Praise for
NARRATIVE HEALING

"Full of exercises accessible to any person with a body and a mind, Lisa Weinert's *Narrative Healing* is sure to help many people on their path to wellness. Lisa reminds us that there is no separation between body and mind, and that if we want to heal either one, we need to work with both."
—Nellie Hermann, creative director at the Program in Narrative Medicine at Columbia University

"Drawing on trauma research and years of experience, Weinert's approach to writing as a method for healing is both powerful and essential. *Narrative Healing* is destined to become a classic text in the mental health arena and beyond, offering a vital resource for anyone seeking to improve their physical, emotional, and mental well-being."
—Amanda Stern, author of *Little Panic: Dispatches from An Anxious Life.*

"*Narrative Healing* is an invitation to write your resistance into recovery and possibility. Lisa Weinert's guidance inspires and catalyzes an inner wisdom that cuts deeper than words. It is an embodied journey back to the self."
—Kerri Kelly, author of *American Detox*

"Lisa Weinert has the rare power to help people find their story. In *Narrative Healing*, she shares her gift for viewing the practice of writing as an act of mindful healing. A must-read for writers, aspiring writers, and those who are still struggling to find their voice."
—Ethan Nicthern, author of *The Road Home: A Contemporary Exploration of the Buddhist Path*

"Profound, inspiring, and accessible, the life-changing therapeutic principles of *Narrative Healing* are essential for anyone on a path of growth, personal healing, and our collective healing. Like a loving friend, Lisa Weinert confidently and compassionately guides us through the process of holding space for ourselves, and listening deeply, so we can feel safe enough to greet, care for, and free not only

our stories but limiting beliefs, identities, and traumas that are diminishing our health and the ability to feel connected and at ease in our bodies and lives. *Narrative Healing* is a path of liberation for all of us."
—Jillian Pransky, author of *Deep Listening*

"Lisa encourages us, as artists of any medium, to look inside and pull inspiration from our own experiences. We each have a story to share, and these prompts and embodied practices are creative gold for all artists."
—Jessica Dimmock, Emmy Award–Winning director

"Lisa Weinert teaches that storytelling is a basic right. *Narrative Healing* is a call to action for all of us to reach inside and ignite the power of our authentic voice in pursuit of our collective healing."
—Nicole Cardoza, founder of Reclamation Ventures, creator of Anti Racism Daily, and author of *Mindful Moves*

"Eloquent and deeply personal, Lisa Weinert bares her soul in this raw and powerful narrative of her own healing journey. A godsend to professionals reeling from the upheavals that have hit the workplace and our lives since 2020, and how releasing our stories unleashes its healing virtues and deepens our sense of social connectedness."
—Kennedy Ihesie, head of Global Diversity & Inclusion at AIG

"As a lifelong mover and professional embodiment teacher, I've seen the power of somatic release to heal trauma firsthand. Lisa Weinert's experience with writing coupled with her dedicated practice in multiple movement modalities, has given her a unique lens in birthing the work of *Narrative Healing*. This is a must-read for anyone on a healing path or looking to actualize their true calling."
—Karla Misjan, movement instructor and Manager of Experience at The Class

"No matter your role professionally, this book will transform your ability to communicate and inspire. Thoughtfully written with insight and compassion, Lisa Weinert's *Narrative Healing* offers a road map to healing and leading in a postpandemic world, where empathy and resilience are the keys to business, creative, and personal success."
—Susan McPherson, author of *The Lost Art of Connecting: The Gather, Ask, Do Method for Building Meaningful Business Relationships*

NARRATIVE
HEALING

NARRATIVE HEALING

Awaken the Power of Your Story

LISA WEINERT

hachette
BOOKS

NEW YORK

Hachette Go, an imprint of Hachette Books
Hachette Book Group
1290 Avenue of the Americas
New York, NY 10104
HachetteGo.com
Facebook.com/HachetteGo
Instagram.com/HachetteGo

First Edition: July 2023

Published by Hachette Go, an imprint of Hachette Book Group, Inc.
The Hachette Go name and logo is a trademark of the Hachette Book Group.

The Hachette Speakers Bureau provides a wide range of authors for speaking events. To find out more, go to hachettespeakersbureau.com or email HachetteSpeakers@hbgusa.com.

Hachette Go books may be purchased in bulk for business, educational, or promotional use. For information, please contact your local bookseller or Hachette Book Group Special Markets Department at: special.markets@hbgusa.com.

The publisher is not responsible for websites (or their content) that are not owned by the publisher.

Library of Congress Control Number: 2023935395
ISBNs: 978-0-306-83039-6 (hardcover); 978-0-306-83041-9 (ebook)

Printed in the United States of America
LSC-C
Printing 1, 2023

This book is for you.

Contents

Part One | Awaken

Part Two | Listen

Part Three | Express

Part Four | Inspire

Part Five | Connect

Part Six | Grow

Introduction

We Share Our Stories for One Reason: We Have To

In my earliest memory of writing, I am nestled under my covers, in a kind of bedsheet cocoon. I am seven, and I am spilling my guts out. I am sending an SOS into the universe. I fill my journal with urgent, exasperated cries like *Help me! Can you believe it?* and *Don't tell anyone but . . .* I am a sensitive and intense kid growing up in New York City with a pile of siblings, high-pressure parents, and great big feelings that I can't always understand or express. I often feel like I am wearing my skin inside out.

When I am writing, I feel heard and seen. My journal is a portal to something larger than myself contained within me, and I am hooked.

Storytelling is the backdrop of my childhood. My mom is an author, and I grew up surrounded by people who earned their living writing books. I learned the ins and outs of literary life alongside learning to eat my greens and make my bed. I'm also from a lineage of women who fought for the right to tell their stories—my Welsh maternal great-grandmother was illiterate and signed her name with an *X*;

two generations later, two of her granddaughters went on to publish books. My Jewish paternal grandmother taught reading at a time when it was radical for white women to work. At every opportunity, she wagged her index finger at me and said, "You must read! They can never take education away." I was taught words matter and that telling my story is a birthright I am bound to preserve and protect.

Writing becomes a daily habit when I'm twelve, and my family moves for the third time in three years; Fifi, my half sister's mother, hands me a black notebook and commands me to write when I am lonely or upset, or happy and excited, or just have something to say. She says, "You can write whatever you want. You can tell made-up stories or write about what you see or about what you feel." She emphasizes this journal is just for me and I don't need to share it with anyone else (but I can share with her if I want to). I am mesmerized.

Fifi is an artist and says, "All great books have a great cover!" We spend the afternoon smearing the journal with a thick coating of oil pastels shaping L I S A in big letters and bold colors, with a rainbow underneath. I feel like I have made my mark.

I start writing daily, reflecting on events of the day and describing my feelings. I write terrible poetry, anonymous love letters, and ambitious short stories. Something about having a reader propels me, and tracking my emotional reality in words makes me feel like I am in charge of my experience.

———

Writing offers an escape from the challenging and at times scary world around me. I write alone, when I think no one is looking. It becomes something like an illicit habit. My journal is my first love, my confidant, my constant companion, and my obsession. Writing takes the edge off.

Along a parallel track, I am a mover; my body is a source of freedom and power. I am called a "tomboy" as a kid. I fantasize about joining the football team and play every sport I am offered. I pursue gymnastics and then dance in high school. When I discover yoga in college, I immediately know it will be a life path. When I pop up into a big heart-opening pose, called Wheel, it is like the universe opens. I feel whole.

Over the years, I commit to a regular yoga practice, but I keep it separate from my writing life. I think the important work of writing comes from my mind and that my body exists to do things for me when it's well and is something to tolerate when it's unwell.

———

My first writing gig is in journalism. I am the editor of my high school and college newspapers and literary journals. I obsess over every headline, every story; I pull all-nighters, skip meals, and drink a lot to hold the seams together. I wear my writing on my exterior, like an identity marker. There's an urgent sense that there's a right way and a wrong way to write, so I wrap myself up in ambition to get by.

In college I experience a mental health crisis, and writing becomes slippery and unreliable. I sink into a severe depression following a few events that overwhelm my system. I feel hopeless, and my body disobeys me; I become clumsy. My legs are like sandbags. I feel trapped in my body. I'm a dean's list student, and I can't think clearly, read or complete simple tasks, or meet deadlines. I cry without warning. I silently sob during an interview for a writing program I'm applying for. The kind professor gently suggests, "Maybe try again next fall." When I try to write, my words separate me instead of soothe me. I create grooves, writing in circles about painful feelings and experiences that lead me further inward and isolate me from the world. I write over and over, *What is wrong with me?* I think I have done something wrong, and my pen is not strong enough to pull me out by itself. The president of the college ignores my pleas to drop out and instead puts me on an enforced medical leave.

I am sent home to fifty-one unopened boxes, an empty apartment, and no place to go. I'm treated like nothing happened and told not to tell anyone. The hardest part isn't what happened; the hardest part is the residue.

My feelings are like tidal waves, and I reach for my pen and paper. I write furious and frantic letters and stories. People who are taking care of me confiscate my writing, saying it's overstimulating. And every day, I try again. With every word on the page, I find myself, then lose myself, and then locate myself again.

———

I survive by wrapping this experience up neatly in a box and burying it. I move, switch schools, straighten my hair, and pretend like it never happened. When I meet people, I edit and parcel out bits of my story. When I graduate, I massage the little interruption in my résumé and doggedly pursue a career in publishing. I work at a major publishing house as a publicist and devote myself to other people's stories for the next decade. I spend my days trying to fix and manipulate every message to secure the right outcome, the right review, or the right story. I start to treat writing more like a weapon or a shield, something I can use to control outcomes. I write pitch letters and emails instead of from the heart. I go to award events and literary parties and decide that if my writing isn't going to win a National Book Award, it isn't worth writing at all.

The more I live in my head, the less I write and the further away I get from my body. I try to squeeze myself into a new story. I focus on pursuing more socially acceptable roles and try to win people over. I get engaged, move to a high-rise apartment, and wear pencil skirts and heels. I feel like I'm wearing a costume that's two sizes too small. I pour alcohol and work over anything and everything to smooth out the rough edges. I go to work, I go out, I go home. I rotate my plans with different acquaintances so I'm not known or accountable to anyone. Life gets harder to manage, and I find myself in precarious situations.

My writing turns on me. It no longer grounds me, because I'm not grounded in my body. My writing is a reflection of my self-perception; I keep punitive lists of what I accomplish every day. I note how much I eat and drink, how much I exercise, how much I write, and how much I read—I have a one-to-five rating system (five meaning great, one meaning unacceptable). There is a sense that if I keep writing it down, I will ultimately get somewhere I want to be. I focus so intensely on hiding my shame, I no longer know my story; I can't express myself authentically in the moment, so I give up my voice and hand the pen over to a hypervigilant unreliable narrator.

I stretch my body beyond its comfortable limits. I run a half marathon. I practice yoga daily. I even try boxing. I try cleanses and go on retreats. I meditate. Nothing makes me feel better because I'm drinking all the time. I negotiate with myself and say, *If I go to a yoga class, it means I am balanced* and *If I keep getting promoted, it means I am happy.* Things start to fall apart. My engagement ends, and I move eleven times in three years. I quit my prestigious job. I think I keep landing on my feet and then spin a story that I am good at dodging bullets. The more uncomfortable I feel, the more actions I take to normalize the discomfort. Eventually I become isolated and bored, and I make the same mistakes again and again.

I think drinking and writing go hand in hand; I think drinking is the lubrication I need to feel inspired. In reality, I'm not writing a single sentence; instead I'm talking about writing while I drink with strangers. I feel indifferent to my life. It is a different feeling than the suicidal feelings or dramatic adventures of the past. Now I feel nothing, like everything is gray. I have a pervasive feeling that nothing matters. It looks like things can only get worse, but then my body wakes me up.

———

In my thirties I suffer another acute medical diagnosis—this time not a mental health crisis but a cancer scare. As I recover, I experience a shift. I learn to listen to my body in a new way. I get sober and begin a journey of recovery. I learn how to let others see me and hear me, and I do the same for them. I start to have a new experience with writing. I write gratitude lists instead of self-punishing ones. Instead of being silenced, I'm encouraged to track and share every emotion and every experience with a safe community who understands, relates, and is available to support me. I meet a kind friend who offers a relaxed ear. When I tell them my wild stories and how good I am at dodging bullets, they cock their head and say, "Maybe one day you won't have to dodge so many bullets." I'm dumbfounded imagining this as a possibility.

Instead of leafing through books I think I should read, I rediscover a joy of reading. I put down morbid thinking and pursue thousands of hours of yoga and mindfulness trainings to learn how to reconnect to my body and understand the stories my body holds. I find a connection to a higher loving force around me. I start inviting my body to the page, pausing, and listening to what is meant to be said rather than barking at the page and ordering it around. In doing so, I start practicing writing with my whole body and listening with my whole self with an aim to connect. I feel whole and I find my voice.

What transpires over the next ten years amazes me. Almost immediately after getting sober, I am invited back as a keynote speaker to the same college I was forced to leave. Soon after, I am invited back as a visiting writer to teach in the very same program that rejected me as an undergrad when I was too depressed (by Anne Greene, the very same professor who years earlier had told me to wait a *little* longer). This same year, I am invited to create the first Narrative Healing program at Kripalu Center for Yoga and Health, a major retreat center, while I am assisting another program. Six months after that, I teach to a packed room of over one hundred people.

As a result of befriending my story and releasing my shame to trusted communities, I am given the opportunity to teach people just like me—and people nothing like me. In doing so, the parts of me that I banished and shamed are returned to me. I develop a new default setting of trust and friendliness in place of distrust and contempt.

I create this program because it is the healing I need, and over the years this work has taken on a life of its own. This process is cyclical and ongoing; there is no end point. Every day I begin again. Every day I need to find my body and find the page. I still use the page to understand the world around me and comprehend my feelings. The writing slows time so my body can catch up, much like a restorative practice. As a result, I'm able to also use the page to connect with others. Over time, I find a sense of belonging to community I never thought possible. I begin attracting and being attracted to open-hearted and grounded people. Writing even leads me to my love. On our very first date, I bring a notebook along. Just when the date feels like it is going well, I am seized with anxiety. I hadn't been on a promising date in years, and I don't know what to do, so I challenge Barry to do a writing prompt. He doesn't miss a beat. He is soon writing away, pen flying across the page, and I know I have met someone who knows how to give me the space I need to collect myself.

I don't think I can adequately describe the joy of witnessing the kind of connections and deep friendships that blossom when people go through this program together. When the pandemic begins in March 2020, everywhere I have been teaching shuts their doors within a week. I immediately start leading Narrative Healing classes and groups over Zoom. Pretty quickly, people assemble from all over the world, coming from Tokyo, Oslo, Tuscaloosa, Manhattan, and Martha's Vineyard—I even have one student Zooming in from a small boat in the Caribbean. I've seen time and time again that after a group session or two, participants treat each other like chosen family. This is a reliable by-product of this kind of whole-body listening and mindful sharing.

———

It's the height of the pandemic, when most of the United States is in lockdown and people are washing groceries with Lysol, running out of toilet paper, and barely leaving their homes. A group I am working with, who were strangers just weeks before and have only known each other on Zoom, hatch a plan to do a Narrative Healing Circle in person. They drive from miles away to meet at one of their homes. I am walking home from Union Square, my glasses fogging up from the mask strapped across my face, when a notification sounds from my phone. A photo pops up of the five of them gathered outside, sitting feet apart, wearing big toothy grins, and sharing stories—an array of cubed cheese and crackers nearby. To this day, they support each other with creative accountability, compassion, and friendship.

This experience is remarkable, but it's not at all unusual. I hear from people all the time that "this work changed my life," "I can finally call myself a writer," or "this is the program I was looking for." Over the years, through this program, I've seen people heal and find joy and a creative spark. Some write books or publish in other ways; I've seen people connect with themselves and others in deep ways and pursue new dreams. The outcomes vary and are often unexpected, but what remains true is this path of embodied writing offers a path to transform after trauma and discover a creative life.

I hope this program is helpful to you.

NARRATIVE HEALING
How It Works

Most writing books, journaling courses, and creative writing programs begin by putting the pen to the page. At Narrative Healing, we begin with the body. We offer a new paradigm for healing from trauma, tapping into creativity, and sharing our stories in the world. The premise here is simple: as we are able to better know our own stories, we are better able to take in the humanity of those around us. My hope is that if we start to listen to the body when it whispers, we won't have to wait for it to scream to hear what it has to say. And we will thus have the capacity to listen to others too.

This isn't a new idea, but it's a new model and framework for addressing creative, spiritual, emotional, and mental blocks to match the world we live in. The Narrative Healing storytelling cycle has clear stages to support maximum nourishment and transformation, leaning on various somatic mindfulness practices and creative prompts. These exercises work both linearly and as a dip-in-and-out tool for prompts and grounding. No prior writing or movement experience is needed. Each part offers various types of mindfulness-based practices and creative prompts that correspond with each stage to meet you where you are. I offer options and modifications throughout; however, only you know what feels comfortable. Please self-adjust and self-pace.

My top intention with this book is to make it as welcoming and accessible as possible. I have done my best to offer a host of modifications and choices throughout to meet you where you are. Still, all of the exercises in this book come from my experience as a heterosexual, cisgender white woman, and I have many privileges I didn't earn, which shape my perspective. This work is deeply personal, and my hope is for you to fully step into your experience. Take what you like and leave the rest. If anything I suggest or say doesn't apply to your experience, modify it in your own way.

The Six-Stage Circle of Narrative Healing

These stages build on one another and work as stand-alone exercises. This journey is intended to accelerate, deepen, and inspire whatever healing journey you are on and uncover the story that needs to be told now. Begin wherever feels intuitive to you. My intention is to offer choices for where to begin so you can seek out the option that will help you best in this moment to reach your goal, wherever you are on your creative and healing journey. You may benefit from reading it through once and then returning piecemeal to exercises and prompts that benefit your creative practice.

1. **Awaken:** Our stories live in our bodies, but they don't speak to us in our native tongue; they speak in the language of the body, through tension and emotion. This step offers gentle, accessible movements, mindfulness practices, and writing prompts to wake up the stories we're holding so we can release their meaning and use their true impact. The result is you'll find your authentic voice in everything you do and say, and you'll also be able to pick up on other people's nonverbal cues. The promise of this stage is to become aware of them, befriend them, and release them through gentle movement.

2. **Listen:** Once you wake up your stories, the next step is to be present with them, pay attention to them, and pause to truly listen to what they have to say. Meditation and other mindfulness practices offer tools to access this kind of listening. The promise of this stage is connection with self.

3. **Express:** The next step is to release these stories onto the page. Writing is a healing practice when approached in this way. Like any other mindfulness practice, the act of

returning without any destination in mind yields dramatic healing results. The promise of this stage is writing to heal and seek meaning.

4. **Inspire**: Writing can be a lonely activity, but you don't need to do it alone. Open yourself up to your muse and spirit, your inner guide, and tap into your creative power. The promise of this stage is a relationship with a higher guide.

5. **Connect**: Sharing your story begins with one chosen, trustworthy person. Using tools to practice trust and choice, receive the radical transformation and healing that comes from sharing your truth with another. The promise of this stage is building trust within and without.

6. **Grow:** Once you have released yourself from the confines of your own lived experience, you can begin to grow beyond your story, engage with the world around you, and enjoy true connection. In the process, you'll find you have the power to heal others too. The promise of this stage is being a source of healing to others and being open to possibility and joy.

WRITING AND TRAUMA

An important note to you about trauma and this book.

While these practices are designed to support trauma healing, they do not replace talk therapy or group work with professionals. I include a number of resources in this book to offer more information about how to find therapeutic help for healing trauma. I recommend working with a licensed trauma-informed practitioner. This book can be used in tandem with professional therapy.

Trauma can happen to everybody; it is part of the life journey. Healing from trauma can also be a part of everyone's life journey. When I'm referring to trauma, I'm referring to a physical phenomenon that happens when the body is overwhelmed by an experience and loses its ability to respond from a grounded place. This might be brought on by an accident, illness, loss, or even something innocuous; it can also be something that lives systemically in the body as part of ongoing oppression or something that was passed on through generations. The effects can be obvious or subtle. The body may lose a sense of time passing and can believe that trauma is happening constantly or intermittently, even when it is no longer experiencing that trauma. It can catch you off guard.

Trauma is relative and subjective. That's why two individuals who grew up in the same family or survived the same accident, or experience, may walk away with different scars and consequences. The body doesn't differentiate between degrees of trauma, because trauma is the experience of the body shutting down, not the magnitude of the event itself. A leading trauma expert, Peter Levine, writes, "When it comes to trauma no two people are exactly alike."[1]

Some of the earliest research on trauma was restricted to focusing on acute catastrophic events like war, violence, physical injury, and assault or abuse. But in recent years, it's become widely understood that trauma can also be caused by ongoing circumstances, systemic racism and intergenerational wounds, abuse, illness, addiction, and types of grief. Depending on a whole host of other factors, like genetics, environment, and other conditions or psychodynamics, trauma can occur with daily events, like a doctor's visit, a fall, or even a hostile email. Individual effects vary. They can show up in anxiety and stress and also physical symptoms, like headaches, stomachaches, insomnia, and other ailments. They also show up in how we experience storytelling. When we experience a traumatic event, our nervous system responds in a variety of ways to offer self-protection—for example, the fight, flight, freeze, or fawn responses. And depending on that response, the stories we experience from ourselves and others are affected accordingly. The conclusion based on many studies is that increasing your awareness of your body and its connection to the stories within can offer a healing path forward.

A writing practice can offer access to this kind of awareness. In this book, I'll describe ways writing can help you heal from trauma. This embodied program provides a method to access hidden, frozen, overactive, or people-pleasing stories that may become disruptive. We can become aware of them, set them onto the page, share them with a chosen listener, and release them into the world. In this way, we integrate past experiences into a new narrative that we author. This process is not a one-time quick fix or a linear path; rather, it's a practice we can turn to again and again each day as old and new memories surface and resurface. Over time, we'll learn to welcome and befriend these memories. The approach is roomy and vast, and there is space for all of them. As a result, through a consistent writing practice over time, you'll have another way to process and digest traumatic experiences, allowing you to move forward confidently with your whole story, whole heart, and whole self to meet the world as it is and as you are.

My offerings are created through a trauma-informed lens, supported by certifications in trauma-informed yoga and therapeutic and restorative yoga. Decades of working with writers as a publicist, editor, and coach on personal stories was also a meaningful training for Narrative Healing, given the deep psychology involved in publishing one's work in the world. I also know this in my own body from my own winding path of seeking trustworthy places, spaces, and people with whom to share my own stories.

The Body and Creative Inspiration

It is through and with your body that you have to reach realization
of being a spark of divinity.
—B. K. S. Iyengar[2]

Your body can be a source of creative inspiration, and the more connected you are to your own bodily flow and energy, the easier it will be for you to create. This holds true for the healing process as well. An embodied writing practice can offer a reliable way to process and heal from traumatic experience. As leading trauma expert and author Resmaa Menakem writes, "We heal primarily in and through the body, not just through the rational brain. We can all create more room, and more opportunities for growth, in our nervous systems. But we do this primarily through what our bodies experience and do—not through what we think or realize or cognitively figure out."[3] So through movement, we'll work together to establish awareness and safety and move into meditation and contemplative practices to truly sit with and listen to the stories that exist within us right now. As we progress through the book, we'll move from inner to outer and begin sharing with the world on the page, with one trusted person and then with groups. In this way, each of us contributes to a ripple effect of healing that's sorely needed in today's world.

Like a yoga class, these writing prompts can be private and personal. You don't need to share anything with anybody. You don't need to make anything. You don't need to be "productive." Your writing can be quiet and humble. Or it can be raw, loud, colorful. You can do this inside with the doors closed or figuratively (or literally) out in the wilderness with nobody around but you and your spirit guides and plant and animal friends. This can be a fearless draft that never needs to be read or seen. And if your goal is to share your stories, this journey will help guide you to know when to share what with whom to maximize your impact, reach, and healing.

———

I started teaching this program in 2014 in an attic studio in New York City with a small group of yoga students and writers. As the program grew, it attracted people who were at some kind of crossroads, at some kind of transition (and who isn't?). I taught artists, writers, trauma survivors, elderly communities, and people living with disabilities, chronic pain, and terminal illnesses. I worked with people recovering from alcoholism and addiction. I worked with a large range of caregivers—doctors, nurses, social workers, therapists, and healing-arts practitioners, seeking ways to nourish themselves and work with burnout. What everyone had in common was that everyone had a story they needed to tell to further their own healing.

When people did this program, they got closer to their truth. New books were born, new careers were launched, and new friendships were formed. I have seen blocked writers write, and people working with illness and disability find joy and relief in creativity. I've seen doctors discover a sustainable form of self-care, memoir writers find clarity, teachers inspire their students. I have seen people who have overcome horrendous personal loss and suffered grave misfortune find joy, meaning, and purpose through telling their stories. This program can work for anybody; no previous writing, yoga, or mindfulness experience is needed. It offers a pathway to heal from trauma, tap into creative inspiration, and forge deep connections with others. That is where the magic really happens. People often experience an emerging clarity and vision as a result of the healing qualities of this program that can lead to unexpected outcomes.

This program is for anyone with a willing heart and open mind; all you need is a desire to listen to yourself and a true willingness to take in what comes up.

BEFORE WE BEGIN . . .

Here are some suggestions for supporting writing as a path to heal from trauma.

Create Sacred and Safe Conditions. Create a quiet, inviting, and safe place; it doesn't need to be fancy or elaborate. Find a place where you can feel relaxed and grounded to access your authentic voice and coax all the other stories out. Take your time attuning to your needs.

Be Gentle. This is deep work, and we'll move slowly. Your body may have stories to tell that are hard to hear. Your body may also be carrying other people's stories—both from your own genetic pool and ones that were picked up along the way. That's okay.

For so many of us, the voice within the body and the voice we use aren't even our own. If you are a Brown or Black body, AAPI, Indigenous, female identifying, LGBTQ, disabled, or living with illness or pain, it's likely your body has been overrun by voices of dominant culture that pervade our media channels, radio, TV, and books. There might be intergenerational trauma or abuse. There may also be stories of resilience and courage. These are valuable lessons that make up you; you are holding them on a cellular level in your muscles and bones.

In these practices, we'll gently wake up different parts of the body, as if we're holding a microphone, amplifying what they have to say. This begins with listening to your body. Some of the stories might be clear as day, like a narrative; others might be a fuzzy frame or even a faint sense.

My hope is that in these practices, you'll begin to find yourself by shaking old stories loose and letting go of any narratives that aren't serving you. These gentle exercises and practices were designed to soothe the nervous system and guide the body from a fight, flight, freeze, or fawn response to rest and restore. Each practice will offer an embodied mindfulness practice followed by an optional prompt.

The idea is that where the body goes, the creative mind will follow. Try one or try them all.

This might lead to the creative gem you've been waiting for, it may release tension, or it might empower you to communicate more effectively with that person you love or even a difficult person. We won't know what our stories have to say until we wake them up.

Everything I'll offer you is an invitation; nothing is required. I'll also offer modifications as we go. Trust yourself. If anything causes discomfort, please don't do it. Welcome all of it. There's no end point or destination. Please move at your own pace. There's no rush. Give yourself permission to approach these pages in whatever manner feels right to you today. If you want to go deeper, go deeper. If you want to skip something, go ahead and skip it. Trust that you know what your body needs right now.

If You Are Writing with Injury

Many writers are working with injury. Please take care of yourself and modify as you go. Common writing ailments include neck stiffness, wrist pain, hand pain, and headaches, in addition to any number of other pains, illnesses, or disabilities you personally are working with. Done over time, mindful movement and quieting practices can help with soothing and strengthening the body and offer preventive care.

Assemble Your Tools and Prepare Yourself

You can do the practices in order or hop around and focus on the ones that stick out to you right away, the "easy" ones that you don't have to think about. It's okay to do the same one again and again and again. The benefits of writing come from doing a consistent practice over time, not from doing as many different prompts as possible. You may find a single prompt keeps your interest.

You may want to record yourself reading these exercises and play them back because some practices suggest closed eyes.

Suggested supplies:
- writing technology of your choosing (notebook and pen, computer, phone, etc.)
- a place where you can be undisturbed
- a timer
- recording device

Suggestions for writing:
- **Time Is Your Friend.** I recommend setting a timer for twenty minutes for each prompt. There's a lot of science that shows that twenty minutes is a magic number when it comes to relaxing the nervous system, so consider these little relaxation breaks or creative savasana. You don't need to write the entire time; you can let your mind wander. Please do not go beyond twenty minutes in one sitting, especially if this is new to you.
- **Pace Yourself.** If you are writing and get an icky feeling, stop. Do not push through pain or unsettling feelings; simply move on or take a break and allow the feelings to settle. Consider returning to one of the practices from Parts 1 or 2 to settle the body and nervous system. Trust your inner compass—it will let you know when you're moving in the right direction.
- **Don't Do This Alone.** Tell someone you trust that you are doing this—to inspire and welcome accountability and support. If you know you're working with trauma or difficult emotions, please consider working with a trained therapist or support group as you write to help process anything that comes up. (See resources at the end of this book.)
- **This Is for You.** Let this practice be a place to dump anything that's blocking you or clogging your thoughts or creative flow.

This practice is just for you. You don't have to do anything with these pages—you can lock them up in your desk drawer, delete the files from your computer, or even burn or otherwise get rid of the physical pages.

- **Stay with Your Body.** Stay close to your body as you write, noticing sensations and feelings. This is where the healing happens.
- **Trust Yourself.** Trust your body, trust your breath, trust yourself. There's no right way to write. You have already done the hard work of showing up. Now make yourself at home and stay awhile.

CONTRIBUTING VOICES

The most inspiring part of Narrative Healing is the incredible people I get to meet while witnessing their growth, joy, and connection. I have invited a cross section of clients, colleagues, mentors, and collaborators along to join us in these pages. Their voices are by no means exhaustive or thorough. They are here to provide a wider range of experiences, wisdom, and perspectives to draw from. Their voices are marked by a light-gray background, and you can find full bios in the end of this book. I hope they resonate with you, and if they don't, I hope you seek out examples that do.

PART ONE

Awaken

AWAKENING

The office is so quiet that the gentle ticktock of her desk clock sounds like an alarm. Looking around the familiar space, I notice a loose pile of papers, including her prescription pad, some medical journals, and a photo of what I assume is her family (a graduation? a birthday?). A few moments later, she returns holding a piece of paper, chewing on a pencil, and slightly shaking her head. "I don't like what I see," she says. As if remembering I am there, she quickly looks up. "I mean, I'm sure it's nothing. It's nothing. But let's check it out."

Unworried, I make necessary appointments and return to my inbox to reply, manage, and execute various author accounts. A few days later, I have an ultrasound. Whatever the doctor's seen, I think I can handle it. Like everything else on my to-do list, I can check this off with a breeze. I don't have any noticeable symptoms.

A week later, I get a call from her office. "You have cancer," she says. "I'm so sorry."

"What?!"

The shock charges through my veins like a bull, thickens my blood, quickens my heart rate, and seals my ears. This story, in the form of a diagnosis, shorts my system. There's no way to spin it. I didn't write this headline. I nod, I swallow, and I hold my breath. I take out my notebook and pen in a gesture of authority, proving my command over the situation. I only ask a couple of questions about logistics.

When I put down the phone, I settle my gaze on a familiar blood-red painting in front of me, as if looking at something I already knew might make time stand still. Just like when I was a child, I believed that closing my eyes would make whatever was happening around me stop.

The first thing I do is text my dog walker, "I may need extra walks in the coming weeks." I make a to-do list. Next, I call my father.

"Dad," I say, "I have cancer." The conversation comes down to the power of that one word repeated again and again, like a spell.

"Cancer?" he says. "You have what? No . . . " He exhales.

"Yes," I say, softer the second time. "Cancer."

"Can't be."

"That's what they said . . ."

"Cancer?" he whispers again.

"I know," I say. "I'm sorry." I can feel the deadly word slither through my body. All I can hear is our breathing.

We move quickly, as if I have a snake bite. Appointments are made. I visit my parents' home. My mother screams and holds me close. I have been bitten, but somehow I infect everyone else too. I feel this is somehow my fault, as if I have the power to edit this story and change its outcome.

Two weeks later, I am at an appointment with a very perky man in a bow tie. He, the surgeon, argues the benefits of removing my entire thyroid. "The only reason to only remove half would be if you were an opera singer," he says with a wink. "Do you have plans to become an opera singer?"

All of my communication skills, every single one of them, float out the window when the doctor enters the room. The white coat and stethoscope have the power to place masking tape over my mouth. I can't summon my voice because my body is frozen. I still have my notebook with me, but I can't write a damn thing. I notice everyone else. My father flexes his jaw. I notice the surgeon's red bow tie and easy laugh. I tuck my voice into a little box deep inside me and keep it locked tight.

I get a second opinion—and a third. Everyone says the same.

I wake up after surgery screaming. They ask me if I have an anxiety condition and give me a pill.

When I get home, there are wrapped boxes of pretty scarves from friends and family, anticipating a scar I will need to hide. Another friend fills my fridge with food. I have dog walks lined up. I am prepared for everything, except how to feel.

Three days later I get a call. My doctor is on the other end. "I have great news! It turns out the pathology report was mistaken. You're cancer-free!"

My mother and best friend come over to celebrate, one holds a bottle of champagne, the other presents a bottle of bourbon. I drink and I sink. A tiny part of me is screaming from the bottom of a well. *How could this be? Why did you take my organ?*

I'm home for the next six weeks and lose my voice on and off. They had said, "You need to stay ahead of the pain." I take all the painkillers. I sleep all day.

The moment I am told I am well is precisely when I realize how sick I am. As I become more honest with myself, I remember previous medical scares, mental health crises, bee stings, surgeries, and a time I was misdiagnosed with spinal meningitis. These incidents all left a great fear in my body but no ability to express it in words. The fear told me to be quiet. It hid in my body and dressed itself up as shame. For whatever reason, *this* medical scare and mind-boggling experience wakes me up. You can call it my moment of grace or line in the sand. My broken body grounds me like an anchor, and the feelings come crashing over me.

There's a Qigong warm-up called "shaking" that's all about shaking the body loose, getting rid of blocked energies, releasing negative thought patterns, and allowing the body to heal. You stand with your feet hip-distance apart, your spine long, and your heels planted on the ground. Then you just shake every part of the body for five minutes without a break. This practice invigorates energy (qi), increases blood flow, improves organ function, and disorganizes the body to let go of habits and toxins. This exercise replicates what animals do after experiencing a trauma: they literally shake to release toxic hormones and regulate the nervous system.

The next few months of my life are something like this: As I heal, I start to shake—well, not literally at first. I start to shake off my assumptions about who I am supposed to be, who I can trust, and what feels safe.

The first thing I do is change nearly everything. With a lot of help, I remove drugs and alcohol from my body. I discover a recovery community and surround myself with teachers and other people who are further along on their healing trajectories than I am, and I mimic them.

Over time, the shake-up starts to grow, and a new clarity emerges. It starts with trying small movements on the floor of my apartment, in the clearing between my sofa and the wall. Summoning what little I can from my decade-long yoga practice, I wriggle around in yoga poses like cobra and child's pose and eventually downward-facing dog. These shapes are my first steps to reclaiming my voice.

On the Concept of Waking Up

Crystal McCreary is a leading yoga, mindfulness, and health educator; teacher trainer; and author of *Little Yogi Deck*.

Every practice offered is invitational, of course. And by that I mean it is all very gentle and very accessible movement. I believe when you give people an "invitation," this means you're encouraging them to opt in or out according to their own instinct or desire or sense of curiosity about having an embodied experience. It also means allowing them to name and give words to the qualities of the sensations they are feeling themselves, as opposed to telling them what they should feel and how it should feel. Invitational language reminds students that they have autonomy over their bodies and therefore have choice and permission to back off or move more deeply into whatever sensations may be arising for them.

When I teach, I make it very clear that we live in a culture, a Western culture, where historically the fallacy of a mind-body split is the prevailing idea. And some may even learn that there is some inherent darkness or evil in the human body. We spend many years in a variety of learning environments that train and direct our minds away from the wisdom of our bodies. And sure, we may have a PE class where we climb ropes and do pull-ups and warm-up drills and exercise-oriented things, and maybe even learn a sport. But those activities are performative and goal oriented, and they're often taught in ways that exclude the valuable opportunity to connect the wisdom that lives in our body to the wisdom in our minds in an explicit way.

Then there's trauma. And it's everywhere and presently spreading like a spider web all the time. Traumatic events are disruptive, and the experience of trauma can often occur as profoundly unpleasant. So when I start offering yoga or an embodied contemplative practice with framing like, "What we're going to do together is begin to integrate and reunify our body-mind, the wisdom that abides in us, and honor and recognize that wisdom as a gift," it becomes clear that this frame isn't necessarily the lens that folks that experience trauma see their body through. Yet I assert that the sensations we experience are messages; sensation is in fact how our body-mind communicates. It speaks the language of sensation and emotion and temperature and tension. So, learning to surf the waves of that adventurous body-mind landscape is part of the journey we are going on. This is an opting-in journey, however, and not always the right journey for everyone all the time. So, part of what we're doing together through mindful movement modalities is learning to decipher the language of our bodies. We endeavor to learn the language that may have been silenced because of trauma, that we avoided listening to because it was really loud or really distracting or it was too subtle and quiet to even discern. Perhaps we just ignored or didn't even pay attention to it in the first place because no one encouraged us to. Trauma-sensitive facilitation reconnects individuals to the possibility of feeling whole in their body-minds again. And this awakening can feel like a rebirth, a remembering of the wholeness that is our birthright.

Our Stories Live in Our Bodies

Have you ever noticed the way your shoulders seem to release after you share a secret that you have been keeping with someone you trust? Or that feeling in the pit of your stomach when you've buried shame? Or how when listening to another person, your eyebrows instinctively rise when something surprises you, your stomach contracts when you hear something scary, or your face falls after hearing something sad? Sometimes slowly and sometimes quickly, the body reacts to how we experience stories. How we create, hold, and experience stories directly corresponds to how we inhabit our bodies. Awakening is something that happens. It's not something we do; it's like breathing.

When we are relaxed, connected, and feeling secure, we are able to move with our stories and respond in an openhearted and flexible way. The stories rise and fall like a breath or a wave; they offer a healing experience. However, when the stories get stuck, silenced, or ignored, they lodge in our muscle tissue, root down in our bones, and stagnate in our blood, making it impossible for us to live full, embodied, and intentional lives.

We are moving bodies of stories. Most of the time, we're only paying attention to the loudest, strongest, and bossiest stories within us; many of our most important stories are frightened, bored, frozen, or *very, very* quiet—even sleeping. Mindfully waking up our sleeping stories—the old ones, the difficult ones, the ones we are avoiding—is a gentle process that requires care and kind, loving attention.

As we awaken our stories and sift through the baggage we are carrying, we uncover the story that needs to be told now.

Before we begin, we must remember that our stories are sleeping for a good reason. They have gone to sleep, and we have left them to protect ourselves from some kind of overwhelming experience. Please trust and respect that. Imagine you were approaching a sleeping child or beloved dog. You wouldn't necessarily shake them or move them around to get them to wake up. You might approach them more gently, offering a loving, gentle nudge or whisper, "Come, now, it's time." We need to move the body with the same tenderness and relax into a state where our stories feel ready—and safe—to come out. That's essentially what we'll do with a combination of gentle movement, breath exercises, contemplations, and prompts for you to choose from.

This tenderness taps into a relaxed place where you can truly listen to yourself and others, unleash your authentic voice, and release the stories you're carrying.

We have become careless with our tender stories; our stories are getting ignored and suffer from neglect, lack of space. And at some point, some of them go silent. We store them away for another time, even when they're important. We're so busy and caught up that we don't know the difference. What happens to all those ignored stories? That text you didn't write? That thing you didn't say? They get zipped up inside your body.

We don't stand a chance at hearing ourselves, expressing ourselves, or listening to others if huge parts of ourselves are asleep and we don't have access to them. That's why this first step is to wake up these stories.

In this section, I'll provide gentle exercises and practices designed to soothe your nervous system and guide the body from a fight, flight, freeze, or fawn response to rest and restore. When we do this, we open up the body to creative flow and foster the conditions to begin a creative practice in the world. This might lead to the creative gem you've been waiting for, it might release a nagging pain in your shoulder, and it might empower you to communicate more effectively with that person you love and a difficult person alike. As you move, the stories will naturally awaken as they are ready.

The Writing Body

Your body is a one-of-a-kind gift for this lifetime, an invaluable, rare archive. Custom-made for you, your body holds the key to creative expression, beauty, and truth, which is always available to you in the moment. Over the past couple decades, science-based research from Harvard's Mind Body Institute and others has shown that there is no separation between the body and the mind. Your brain is in your gut, your grief is in your lungs, and your senses are on your fingertips. There are so many ways to express this, and they all add up to one indisputable fact: we are one, and each part is communicating with the others all day long. The way we are with our bodies impacts how we are on the page.

In the West we live in a culture that is constantly telling us our bodies don't matter and that everything is in our mind. It can be difficult to admit and accept that your body is precious. When we do refer to our bodies, it's usually because we're being told something is wrong—it's too big, too small, too sick, too old, or the wrong color, shape, age, or gender.

It's a tall order for many of us in Western culture to even admit we have a body. We are so committed to the idea that our bodies are somehow separate from us—separate from the mind, our desires, and even our lives. Ironically, the more successful, in a capitalist sense, you are, the more you think your body doesn't matter. Even artists, creators, and writers believe we are walking heads, as if everything that matters exists between our ears.

As a writer, your body is your instrument, whether you are writing by hand, typing, tapping, or dictating. Imagine the body for a moment when it writes. Here is a typical posture: a torso folds forward, the head hangs down, the spine rounds. The shape is an exaggeration of the human condition. The world is constantly dragging us down and into ourselves, through forces like gravity, aging, emotional weight, and even the news. It looks something like this: hunched over a desk with a computer or notebook for hours, barely breathing, barely moving. If you removed the desk and writing technology, you might think this individual was hiding from something. We associate this position as a "thinking position"; it also implies that somehow all thought can be dumped straight from the skull to the page as the head leans closer and closer to the desk. But since our stories live in our bodies, if we don't move, we lose access to huge chunks of creative inspiration. We need to learn how to expand and open up to activate our creativity and receive inspiration.

The Language of the Body

If in doubt of where to begin, start with your own body!
Move it in whatever capacity is available to you or
that lights you up or inspires you or feels accessible.
The story will come.

—Crystal McCreary

Your body is telling you stories all day long. It speaks in the form of sensation, temperature, tension, desire, hunger, ease, pleasure, disgust, joy, illness, curiosity, pain, restlessness . . . These sensations are like little poems. They are like a map. And yet it's hard to pick up on any of these nuances because most of the time our bodies are asleep, stressed, or trying to fit into a mold to please others.

In order to understand the precious stories our bodies are telling us, we need to speak the language of the body. Many of us don't become aware we have a body until it is screaming—in pain, in shock, in despair, or when a doctor or loved one points out we need to pay attention to it. In these practices, we'll learn to become more sensitive to softer voices so we can respond earlier with care.

In this section, we're going to move, stretch, and awaken the body with simple, accessible mindfulness practices. We'll build body awareness and foster relaxation. It's a way of inviting your whole self to the page.

Writing and the Nervous System

The nervous system has one job: to keep us safe. It has four gears it can move in to protect us (fight, flight, freeze, or fawn) and speaks to us in stories, sensations, temperatures, tensions, and emotions. The nervous system is like the ultimate inner editor, forever filtering and dressing up the stories that come in and out to protect us. Whatever state you are in will completely determine the stories you tell and hear. You can think of the nervous system as the format, genre, pace, tone, voice, speed, lens, filter, and temperature.

If our nervous system perceives danger, it will filter stories to inspire us to fight, flight, freeze, or fawn. These stories will be shaped in different ways depending on what the optimal response for safety is. For example, if the best option is to fight and take opposition head on, we'll perceive stories as dangerous, and we may argue or react. If our nervous system thinks the best response is to flee or run—for example, as if a direct threat is coming our way—we may avoid the problem or disappear. There are also times when the safest thing to do is fawn, or *conform*, to find likeness with a group, even if we don't fully understand or agree. We see this all the time with performative, well-intentioned, but empty social justice actions on social media and with false flattery.

As trauma therapist, yoga teacher, and somatic therapist Eva Ludwig says,

> What informs our brain as to what might be perceived as dangerous is as much socially constructed as it is learned through personal experience. For instance, how did we learn to fear people in Black bodies? In Trans bodies? In Fat bodies? Why does one feel the need to cross the street or protect oneself from a Black man in a hoodie? Or why does one feel the need to create a big performance of what they think is allyship by posting a black box on social media or in placing minoritized folks on a pedestal as if to prove to self you're not racist, or sexist, or agist, or fatphobic, or transphobic, or homophobic. It is all forms of dysregulation.

Writing and Safety

It's not always possible to be safe. We live in a chaotic and dangerous world full of real threats, violence, and oppression that threaten each of us in different ways. However, it is always possible to move toward feeling regulated and seeking inner peace and serenity in the moment. As psychologist Dan McAdams says, "Although we can't control everything that happens to us, we can control the stories that we tell about ourselves."⁴ When you feel fully regulated, grounded, and safe in your body, then your nervous system can shift into rest and restore. Then it is wired to connect, seek sameness, listen, and also to befriend, to love, to create. This is the state our nervous system needs to be in to truly practice deep listening, to be creative and inspired, and to access our authentic voice.

Writing can help you slow down, process, and develop an intimate friendship with yourself.

Stories are information, emotions, and plots that stem from our nervous system—the way we process, digest, and share this material determines our basic health and ability to connect to others. Narrative comes in many forms. It can be expressed in motion, breath, words; it can be vocalized, sung, and felt. Our nervous system is designed to respond to stories as they come our way. It's part of our built-in survival tool kit.

We seek and create meaning through our stories. It's how we share our values, beliefs, identities, desires, fears, and needs, and it's how we inspire each other to feel, take action, and change. In this book, we will work with a writing practice to aid this digestion and maintain the maximum nourishment from each moment.

On storytelling and healing, from Crystal McCreary:

> The most unexpected and beautiful gift that yoga gave me was recognizing the stories that live in my body. There are moments of insight that ebb and flow with imagery or language during practice that can, like pieces of a quilt, be woven together to tell a wise or elaborate tale. I have experienced enough ahas and exhales to witness my wounds slowly and

eventually getting healed as I one day wake up and suddenly remember that I once had stage fright, or paralyzing anxiety that no longer exists. It's a wavy, almost magical process.

Over the course of my life, I've learned through embodied contemplative practice to trust. I have faith that simply paying attention and honoring myself by caring for my body and mind in equal measure will eventually lead to something special.

Welcome

Greeting yourself with pleasure will clear a path to finding your voice.

Imagine you are driving a car with a spacious back seat. There's plenty of room for all the different versions of you—the crying infant, the angry teenager, the victim, the menace, the thrill seeker, the joyful one.

Use your imagination and turn around. Observe the back seat. Who's here with you? Which parts are present? Welcome all the parts.

Write it!

Describe the different parts of you who are present. What are they wearing? How old are they? What are their characteristics?

Arrive

Once you have fully arrived, you can inhabit a new space in which you are willing to receive the story you're meant to.

Find a comfortable seat or lie down.

Take five deep breaths with the sole intention of arriving here and now. You may consider placing a hand on your heart and a hand on your belly while using the following mantra:

On the inhale silently say, "I am," and on the exhale silently say, "Here." Inhale. "I am." Exhale. "Here." And so on for a few minutes.

Write it!

Write the story of how you got here.

Create Conditions

When you are taken care of, you are better able to care for your creative practice.

Take a moment to check in with yourself.

Do you feel safe?
Are any parts feeling uncomfortable?
Are you hungry?
Are you thirsty?
Are you tired?
Are you restless?
Are you cold?
Are you hot?
Do you have to use the bathroom?
Are you wearing comfortable clothes?
What else is on your plate today?
Is anything causing you tension or stress personally?
    Professionally?

Please take a moment to tend to yourself in any way you need to increase your comfort.

Write it!

What needs do you usually tend to?
What do you usually ignore?

Warm Up the Writing Body

Motion is lotion and will loosen up stuck
stories.

Find a comfortable seat and take a few deep breaths.
Imagine there's a bowl of soup resting on your pelvis.
Rock your pelvis forward and back just enough to slosh the soup
    around without spilling it.
If you want to add on and if it is accessible to you, you can move
    to all fours.
Place your hands beneath your shoulders and your knees beneath
    your hips.
Spread your fingers and press down between your thumb and
    index finger.
Press down through your shins and top of your feet.
Breathe in and round your spine.
Breathe out and extend your belly, arching your back.
Breathe in and round, exhale and arch, and repeat five times.

Modification for lying down

Lie down and connect; feel the support beneath you.
On an in breath, gently tuck your pelvis, and on an out breath,
    arch your back. Continue in a gentle rocking with your
    breath.

Find Your Seat

Your voice rises when you take your seat in the world.

Most of us are pretty familiar with the concept of sitting down. For many Americans sitting for long periods of the day isn't a choice, it's a lifestyle; on average adults in the United States spend eleven hours a day sitting.

In this book when I say "sit down"—or "take a seat," or "find your seat"—I'm talking about something different. In yoga and meditation, "taking a seat" is about taking the resting position that is most supportive for your breath so that meditation is possible. For our purposes, we're interested in the position that will maximize your ability to find your voice and access creativity, which is the same as a meditative seat. Once your breath comes easily, so will your voice and creative expression. There's no one way to do this. Every moment, every day, you have choices; at any point you may choose a different seat. In meditation, the purpose of sitting is to find a relaxed position for breath, energy, and creativity to flow through. Pay attention to what your body needs in this regard as you take your seat.

Here are a few suggestions for sitting to choose from:

- Sit on a chair with your feet firmly on the ground.
- Sit cross-legged on the floor with a cushion.
- Sit on bent knees on a block or cushion.
- Lie down on the floor or bed or sofa in a way that your spine can settle and you feel comfortable. Offer yourself any other props that might help you feel more comfortable, like a pillow, towel, bolster, sofa, or bed—you name it.

Write it!

What would it feel like to find your seat in the world?

Find Your Footing

You can't know where you're going until you
know where you are.

Our feet can be thought of as the most willing part of the body, and yet we ignore them and rarely offer them praise. For some of us, they go everywhere our mind tells them to go. They are a living archive of where we've been. Yet most of us are completely disconnected from our feet. We spend time in shoes all day long, which desensitizes, softens, and in some instances squishes or pinches our feet. This blocks our connection to the earth and our sense of being comfortably connected to the world around us.

Increasing sensitivity in your feet will increase your awareness in all areas of your mind and body and connect you to the earth beneath you. Enliven the root of your body and reconnect yourself to the ground.

Try it!

Place a tennis ball, golf ball, or small stone or crystal on the ground. (If you have some kind of foot roller, you can use that. A simple rolled-up towel can also work.)

Now step on the support lightly and feel your weight moving into the object and the object moving into your foot.

Take five deep breaths.

Breathe in this position, and then move the object to another area of your foot and continue.

Next, move to a third and final area.

Breathe here.

Now, do the same with your other foot.

When you have done both feet, stand and notice your feet on the ground.

Spread your toes and press your feet down.

Modification for sitting or lying down

Flex and point your toe and focus on the sensation in your ankle.

If this is not available to you, focus on any part of your body that is making a connection with the ground and breathe into that sensation, or use your imagination to connect with the ground.

Write it!

Describe your feet. Where have they been? How do they feel?

Set Aside Expectations

Removing expectations makes room for a new experience.

Fear is one of the greatest obstacles to creative freedom. Fear of the blank page, fear of what others will think, fear of being ridiculed, fear of being pitied. Fear can manifest as tension and anxiety, and it can physically appear as a gripping in the body, stomachaches, and irritation. A mindfulness meditation can offer an alternative way to begin a practice.

Try it!

Find a comfortable seat and take a few rounds of breath.

Imagine you are lying down on your favorite spot and gazing up at a beautiful blue sky with nothing to do but watch clouds float by.

Recall everything that has happened before you got to this page. This could be from today, or perhaps earlier than that. There's no rush.

Look up at the sky and imagine each cloud is a memory. Let each one roll by, the way clouds do. Allow them time to float by. Do this for about a minute or two.

Now, check in with your body. How does it feel to be breathing in your body? Are you comfortable? Do you need to make any adjustments?

Next, imagine everything you expect to happen in the following pages (or insert whatever you are having expectations about).

Notice how you feel about the word *expectations*.

Use your imagination to return to your favorite spot and look up at the imagined sky again. This time let each cloud represent an expectation. Let each one pass, slowly and gently, one by one.

Look at them with the same intensity and level of interest with which you might look at a familiar commercial on TV—passively.

Be here for a few minutes. Please don't rush. Stay as long as it takes for you to acknowledge your expectations.

Write it!

Free write for five minutes, without expectations. Write anything that comes up, even if you only write, "I have nothing to say." The idea is to put the pen to paper, fingers to keyboard, or words to dictation and keep going.

Find the Breath, Meet the Moment

The fastest way to find the present moment is
to find the breath.

Treat this breath like you are swinging on a swing. On an inhale, let
the breath fill you up and swing high, and as you are swinging down,
exhale.

Try it!

Breathe in for a count of six.
Hold for one count.
Breathe out for a count of eight.
Repeat three times.

Contemplate it!

What has changed? What has remained the same?

Take Up Space

Take up space in your body to take up space on the page.

When was the last time you stood with purpose for any extended period? The writing body is in a natural forward fold. It faces down and in. It's rounded and hunched over. Gravity pushes us down; the weather can push us down; news can push us down; trauma can push us down. Standing or sitting upright with purpose is a radical posture in opposition to the forces around.

Being upright with purpose is a radical way to hold your body and also to live your life. It takes courage to feel your full length. In yoga, we call this mountain pose, literally taking on the quality of the mountain. This is the position of truth.

Try it!

Try this seated, lying down, or standing.

> Separate your legs, hip distance.
> Press down with your feet.
> Spread your toes and firm your muscles.
> Lift your chest and drop your tailbone.
> Lift your shoulders up, back, and down.
> Extend your arms alongside you.
> Lift your heart.
> Spread your shoulders.
> Rest your chin parallel to the ground.
> Set your gaze ahead toward the horizon.
> Take five breaths.

Modification for lying down

Lie down on your bed, or a mat, and stretch out in every direction that you can.

Reach and move your limbs, like you're making a snow angel.

When you feel you are making your biggest shape, take five breaths.

Modification for sitting

Seated on your chair, reach out in every direction.

Use any part of your body that is available to you and reach in different directions.

You might use your arms, fingers, toes, or tongue—or your imagination.

When you feel that you are as stretched as you can get, take five breaths.

Write it!

What does it feel like to be tall?

What does it feel like to be small?

Slow Down

Awareness happens one step at a time.

Think for a moment what it really feels like when you shoot off a text while you're walking. Recall what it feels like when the person you are talking to over dinner is distracted on their phone or caught up in their thoughts. We hold our breath or harden and round our shoulders to ward off a fight, either with someone else or perhaps with information itself. This becomes our uniform. Awareness doesn't only happen in a yoga studio or self-help book. It happens while you are going about your daily life, one step at a time.

Try it!

Next time you move to the kitchen, move half as fast.

Wait for the green light to cross the street. (This might be mostly for city mice.)

Wait your turn when you're put on hold by customer service.

Look for something new on your morning commute.

Don't rush for the bus/train/car.

Do one thing at a time.

Write it!

What are five more ways you can slow down?

Process

Trauma lives in your body. You can release it.

To protect ourselves in the moment, we might hold on to traumatic stories and freeze them in time. We can store them in our bodies, and if we don't process or release them, we may end up reliving these stories over and over and over again.

Trauma lives in our bodies in the form of tension. The higher the emotional intensity of the trauma, the more tension that can get trapped. This impacts our writing lives in multiple ways. It influences the stories we think we need to tell and can also create a number of physical symptoms, like lower back pain, stomachaches, and tension-related symptoms.

You probably know what yours are if you're reading this book.

This practice is a quick way to offset tension and stress throughout the body. You can do this practice all day long.

Try it!

Take a few breaths to center yourself.

On an inhale, take one long breath in and tighten every muscle you can. Close your fists and squeeze your eyes, your thighs, your toes. Bring your shoulders up to your ears. Squeeze everything for five counts. Then let it all go with a sigh.

Repeat this three more times.

Write it!

What did you squeeze? What did you let go?

Practice for Difficult Feelings

You can regulate your body so you can be useful to yourself and others.

One thing we can count on is that change is constant. Some change will lead to ease and some change might lead to increased challenge. This can be caused from internal or external factors; our sense of safety can turn on a dime due to the weather, a piece of news, a phone call, or feelings of pain or discomfort, even when our own body isn't touched. There's a concept in medicine that when someone loses a limb, they still have sensations from that limb, even after it is amputated. It's called phantom limb pain. The way we experience pain from trauma is very similar; we can feel the pain even long after the actual event is no longer happening.

The question becomes this: How do you soothe and work with these phantom traumas? How can you regulate your body so you continue to be useful to yourself and others?

I had the great fortune of attending beloved meditation teacher Pema Chodron's final address at Omega Institute in the spring of 2022. It was an incomprehensibly baffling week marked by senseless gun violence in Uvalde, Texas, and Buffalo, New York. Over the course of the weekend, her teachings vacillated from the collective wounds to personal stories. The five hundred people gathered each brought their own story, and baggage, as well as a collective, complex grief.

Pema led us through this "handshake" practice, which feels especially resonant for writers. Let's try it with something small.

Try it!

Find a comfortable seat and take a few rounds of breath.

Bring to mind a small incident that is bothering you—try to think of something relatively easy to work with, like someone cutting in front of you or feeling lonely.

Hold your two hands out in front of you.

Imagine that one of your hands represents whatever is troubling you. With your other hand, gently stroke it and metaphorically offer it whatever you need.

For example, if you are working with loneliness, then offer sympathy, companionship, and anything else you think the situation might benefit from.

You can try this with any situation in your life or in the world that is troubling you or even annoying you. Something like bad traffic, a broken remote, canceled plans, or a heartache or grief. You can also apply it to a sticking point in your writing, like writer's block or when having trouble writing about challenging emotions. It's a way of offering yourself a way to soothe, accept, and care.

You can do this anytime, anywhere.

The Earth Has Your Back

We are all connected and supported by the great big safety net holding us all—the earth.

It's hard to feel connected when you're living with trauma. Traumatic experiences can lead you to isolate from social situations and feel lonely and also separate from your whole story. It's hard to remember you're not alone.

One way to connect with this feeling of support is to find the earth. Even when you might feel alone, one way of reminding yourself that you are not is to lean into the ground. It's always there. Try seeking this existing support as you move through your day. You can feel the support of the earth from all the structures around you, including walls, desks, keyboards, and other surfaces.

Try it!

Find the earth quality within reach. If you don't happen to be outside right now, try leaning against the back of your chair or against a wall or car seat. You can find relief and support in whatever solid object is near you.

You can also feel the ground by using your imagination. Bring to mind the mud of the earth, the dry desert, the grass, the plants, anything that arises.

The earth is always supporting you.

Find Your Wrists

Flexible wrists foster a flexible story.

As you write your story, you move between past, present, and future. As your feelings and thoughts meld on the page, you can integrate your experience. This feeling of integration is more powerful when you feel it with your whole body, not just the page.

Integration will also help recenter scattered ideas and thoughts and recenter your energy. Added benefits include improved circulation in your hands and arms and relaxed tension in your shoulders. This is an effective preventive measure against stiff joints, carpal tunnel syndrome, and other common writing injuries.

Try it!

Interlace your fingers into a gentle fist and roll your wrists in one direction for three breaths. Then move in the other direction. Try to move in a smooth, even way, like you're moving through molasses. It doesn't matter if you move in perfect circles or figure eights; what's important is that you move with ease.

Now, interlace your fingers the other way and move your wrists in both directions on the other side.

Write it!

Write a gratitude list for your wrists.

Create Space

We need to make room in our bodies to make
room for our stories.

In her slim book on feminism, *We Should All Be Feminists*, Chimamanda Ngozi Adichie writes, "We teach girls to shrink themselves, to make themselves smaller. We say to girls, 'You can have ambition, but not too much.'"[5]

Who among us hasn't felt at some point that we needed to make ourselves smaller, thinner, lighter, quieter, less of that or more of this? One way or another, we're taught to get small, play it safe, play the part. Playing small is also a survival instinct when we're experiencing trauma. The body rounds and gets compact, like a ball. As you heal and get stronger, you can expand and experience your creative potential.

Try it!

Find a standing or seated position and stretch your arms out wide, like an airplane. Now widen your knees, or if you're standing, widen your stance. Take a few breaths there, stretching out in every direction.

Notice where your ribs are and avoid arching or rounding your back; instead lengthen your spine.

Modification for lying down

If you're in bed, widen your legs or arms, or simply look out.
Take up as much space as you can.
Wherever you are, stay there for five deep breaths.

Write it!

What does it feel like to expand?

Your Body Is Always Telling a Story

> Rabbi David Ingber is a writer, the founding rabbi of Romemu, and the senior director of Jewish Life at 92Y.

It all begins in your own sensory experience. Growing up, I was very disembodied even though I was an athlete. I really wasn't aware of the body as a place where you live and where you begin from. As a young man, I was under the tutelage of a master therapist and a yogi and became aware that our body is telling a story all of the time. I began to become aware of the experience of my body and how it changed my mind state and my emotional state. I began to notice how my voice changed and my breathing changed when I was more embodied or more present in my body. Tracking what was happening in my body became very important. As I grew in my spiritual practices, it became clear that the most basic place to begin from is the body.

So when I'm teaching, first and foremost, I attune myself to my own body. My teachings are received differently when I am in my own body versus when I'm disconnected from it. The quality of my voice is different, and the way it lands is different depending on whether I'm in a very manic or frantic state of mind; I can use that awareness to slow myself and also the group down and attune them. When you're teaching it's really an attunement that's happening.

Write it!

Write about a time your voice felt aligned with your body or a time it did not.

Embody Your Voice

Where you speak from changes how you are heard.

Finding your voice can mean many things. You may find your voice on the page, in conversation, or within. One way to navigate your voice is to become more aware of where it resides.

Science, myths, medicine, and spiritual traditions all explore how stories resonate with specific purpose. Your body can also change the way a word sounds and influence its meaning. Where a sound comes from changes the way we hear and understand the meaning of the word and even the intention of the speaker.

You don't have to be a speech therapist or therapeutic voice coach to know this; we know this intuitively. Look at the following descriptions and observe what associations or judgments you have with each sound.

Tinny:

Nasal:

High-Pitched:

Breathy:

Monotone:

Husky:

Ringing:

Matter-of-Fact:

Small:

Strident:

Sweet Honey:

Consider which part of the body you think the voice comes from and what the tone means. On a nervous system level, do any make you feel safe? Unsafe? Settled or unsettled? Next time you are speaking, notice and reflect on where the voice is coming from and what that tells you. You can incorporate this into your writing as you develop characters or dialogue.

Beneath the Surface

Relax your face to relax your thoughts.

Your face is your window to the world. Offering it loving care will set the tone for all your interactions, both internally and externally. How you treat yourself is how you treat your story.

We're all carrying huge amounts of tension in our faces because of the screen time most of us are subjecting ourselves to. Did you know your face freezes when you look at screens? This adds to any tightness you're already holding and can cause headaches and jaw pain and limit your perspective.

Try it!

- Relax your forehead: Create a paddle with your index and middle finger. Press this paddle gently into the middle of your forehead and spread out toward your temples. Do this a few times.
- Relax your jaw: Begin at your chin and move the finger paddle in a circular motion up your jawline to your ears. Tug gently on your ears and repeat.
- Relax your neck: Take your dominant hand and gently grab the nape of neck and tug lightly, as if you are picking up a puppy. Tug gently a few times.
- Relax your scalp: Make a cone with your fingers, and place your fingertips on the top of your skull. Extend your fingers in all directions and slide them around the circumference of your skull, making a spider-leg shape with your hands. Repeat a few times as you like. Next, bring your fingers to the top of your skull and begin to bounce your fingertips against the top of your skull. You can also press down and make circular motions into your skull. See what your skull, hair, and fingers need.

A Practice for Grief and Sorrow

Loss, grief, and sorrow are unavoidable, but suffering through them is avoidable.

Trace your collarbone with your index finger. Feel for the hollow space beneath your collarbone, and move your finger until it meets the soft place close to where your shoulder begins. There's a pressure point there that's associated with your lungs and can relate to feelings of grief. Lightly press down and breathe deeply in and out. As you tap into your own feelings, it will expand your ability to feel compassion for others.

Write it!

Write about anything that comes up.

Shake

When the world feels like too much, you can always shake it off.

This practice is a version of the Qigong exercise I wrote about earlier. It can be uplifting, offer a feeling of lightness and happiness, and generate ideas and fresh perspective. It also helps increase circulation and loosen joints.

Try it!

Begin standing, sitting, or lying down with your feet hip-distance apart, or wider, and let your arms dangle by your sides.

Slightly bend your knees and let your shoulders drop.

Gently tap your heels, letting them lift and lower onto the floor with a bounce.

Begin flapping your hands around and shaking your arms.

Move your hips side to side.

Shake your whole body! Shake everything you can shake!

Continue shaking for approximately five minutes, or the length of your song. Find your own rhythm. There's no wrong way to do this! Shake whatever you can.

When you feel done, return to your original position, bring a hand to your belly and a hand to your chest, and feel the energy you created.

Write it!

Write about what that felt like.

The Best Protection Is No Protection

As we become better aware of the stories we're holding, we may no longer need to defend ourselves as much because we are no longer protecting an illusion. We can soften, de-escalate tension, and embrace our own vulnerability. This vulnerability becomes our greatest defense.

Write it!

Write about a time your vulnerability was your greatest strength.

Outward Instinct

Lift your chest; spark your heart.

Standing hunched over with your hands in your pockets might be a wise way to walk outside on a cold day or react to difficult news or grief, but it's not very conducive for wholehearted communication. If we walk around protecting our chest all the time, we can't fully access our feelings or speak from our heart. This exercise is a powerful one for the writing body. It asks you to counter the natural instinct to go inward and crack open your heart using your hands.

This warming sequence can be a great way to support back health and is a preventive exercise for wrist and forearm injury.

If you have any shoulder, arm, or hand discomfort, skip this one.

Try it!

- Stand one arm's distance away from an empty wall that has some space around it (avoid columns, framed artwork, or mirrors). You can do this seated or lying down, placing your hand against any surface (like a book or tray).
- Slightly bend your knees.
- Reach your right arm toward the wall, slightly higher than your shoulder.
- Move your shoulders up, back, and down. Lengthen your arm and firmly press your full palm into the wall and take up to fifteen cycles of breath.
- When you're ready, repeat on the other side.

After stretching both wrists, pause and bring your hands to the body or in a prayer position and ask for guidance on what direction to take with your writing practice today. Acknowledge your own efforts, and devote the benefits of this practice to your future story.

Lift Your Legs, Release Your Past

The past is never dead. It's not even past.
—William Faulkner[6]

It's commonly understood that old emotions and relationship pain and baggage live in the lower body—the hips and legs. In order to release them, you need to release your legs. This gentle inversion will relieve stress, calm the mind, open the heart, and alleviate tension.

To set up for this posture—legs up the wall—you'll need a wall, chair, or firm pillow.

Place a folded blanket about six inches away from the wall.
Sit on the floor with your feet on the ground and your left side
     parallel to the wall.
Roll onto your back, curl up into a fetal position.
Wiggle your way toward the wall and slowly lift one leg and
     then the other onto the wall.
Place a pillow under your head.
Close your eyes or place an eye pillow over your eyes and
     breathe. As you breathe, your legs will relax.

You can do this same setup with a chair or lying down on a bed with a firm pillow under your calves.

Express gratitude for all the places your legs and feet have taken you. Let the legs empty everything they've carried. Go inward. Let go of any active energy.

Stay for at least one minute and up to twenty minutes.

When you're ready to come out of this, begin deepening your breath and *slowly* rise from the floor to return to a comfortable seat. Allow yourself a full minute to rest and recalibrate after this deep pose.

Nap-Asana

Rest is a powerful form of self-love, reclamation,
and renewal.

In recent years, the study of rest has become one of the most popular
subjects, ranging from Yoga Nidra to restorative yoga, yin yoga,
sleep clinics, and sleep tanks. As an overworked, sleep-deprived culture, we need a lesson in nap time. Tricia Hersey, the founder of the
Nap Ministry, which is devoted to supporting rest as a form of resistance and liberation, writes, "My rest as a black woman in America
suffering from generational exhaustion and racial trauma always was
a political refusal and social justice uprising within my body."[7]

In yoga this practice of resting and going inward is referred to as
pratyahara practice. Yoga offers various practices and poses that
instruct one to go inward, reducing stimulation and encouraging
inner presence and potent relaxation. For our purposes, we'll be
imaginative and flexible and consider a word closer to *catnap*. The
idea is to reclaim what rest looks like within your lifestyle. Seek out
an extra twenty minutes to rest in the afternoon—take a longer
shower or bath, walk slower, sit on the couch an extra three minutes.
Create time for rest.

Try it!

Lie down on the floor, on a mat, on a bed, or on a sofa. Place any
kind of support that appeals to you and is available (like a pillow,
rolled-up towel, or bolster) under your knees, and have a similar support under your head. You may choose to add pillows, blankets, or
an eye pillow. Your eyes can be closed or gently gazing above.

Set the intention of receiving the benefits of this practice. Ask for something you want to receive. May this practice help you be more willing and able to receive the support you will need, perhaps from a friend, an editor, a reader, a healer, or a stranger on your path who may have the nugget of wisdom you didn't know you needed. Sometimes the wisdom we need comes from an outside source.

Write it!

List five ways you can rest.

PART TWO

Listen

HEART IN HAND

Delia Ahouandjinou's hands float just above my body, gliding from my feet to the crown of my head. I'm lying on a cot, and it's just the two of us in this small studio. In the corner of the room, a pink vase holding a few lavender stems rests on a delicate wooden table. A breeze wafts through the window; the white linen curtains cast dancing shadows on the blurred black-and-white photograph of a torso that hangs on the wall.

"Take a few deep breaths," Delia says. "Try to relax."

I hear a siren and a man yelling from the street three stories below, the usual noise of downtown Manhattan. The sounds hit me like pelting rain, and my body stiffens and jolts.

I've been feeling on edge, like something's wrong. From the outside, it doesn't look like anything is wrong. I have a job, an apartment, friends. Yet I have stomachaches and headaches every day. I feel jumpy, worried, and irritable. Out of sync. I recently saw a doctor about these mysterious symptoms. They checked my vitals and ran extra blood tests just to be safe. I'm willing to try anything, which is why I'm here today. Delia is a manual therapist trained in multiple modalities, including osteopathy, Reiki, craniosacral therapy, and somatic emotional release. I want her to tell me what's wrong and how to fix it.

My eyes are closed. I feel heat, an energy. I can't quite tell what Delia is doing. Her palms hover over my heart. The area around my lower ribs (*my sternum?*) feels enlivened, electric.

"There is a lot of tension in your chest, around your heart," Delia says. "I'm going to focus there today."

I close my eyes. *What is wrong? Why is she focusing on my heart?! None of my symptoms have anything to do with my heart, do they?* I worry something else is wrong, something I haven't even thought of yet. I try to keep my attention focused on the electric feeling of Delia's energy, which soon settles into a warm, soothing sensation, like sunlight.

As I relax, I see images, as if I'm watching a movie. I'm transported back to the summer before college. I'm working as a dishwasher at a conference center in New England. It's the summer I start drinking daily, the summer I decide lime in a diet soda constitutes a meal. I feel wild and free, and I'm slowly poisoning myself. It's the summer I start passing out.

"What is happening, Lisa?" Delia asks. "What do you notice? What are you aware of?"

I shift a little and come back into the room. There's a faint smell of sage.

"I see a barrel-chested teenage boy with a shock of red hair. I see a young woman with kind green eyes, blond hair . . . I hear music blasting. Madonna? There's commotion." I see myself lying on the ground in jean cutoffs, hiking boots, and an apron on the dish room floor. That was the first time I fainted. I pass out again at a party and then later in my room.

"That sounds intense," Delia says. "Is there more?"

"I see a nurse with papery skin and short gray hair, maybe in her sixties. She holds my arm too tightly and takes my blood pressure. Everything is normal, but she sends me to the hospital to be safe." I feel a tightness in my gut and am quiet for a while.

"Is there more?"

"I'm in the hospital. I see bright lights, white, and metal. I'm on a cot. I'm cold."

"Do you remember anyone else there?"

I pause, scanning this large room. "I'm alone. No, there's a doctor. They run a lot of tests and ask questions I don't know the answers to."

"How does Lisa feel?" Delia asks.

"Worried." They can't figure out what is wrong with me, so they give me a black plastic box called a heart monitor. It's the size of a pack of cigarettes, and they tell me to wear it for two weeks. Just to be safe. I wear it like a chunky charm necklace. It's a party trick—everyone wants to be around me. I can connect in a way I never could before. I drink even harder than usual, fantasizing it might be the last time and wondering if I deserve this attention.

My eyes are still closed; something shifts. I feel pressure on my chest, like Delia is pressing her finger against my heart, though I know she isn't touching me.

"What happened next? How does Lisa feel?"

Feel? I'm not sure. I keep seeing images. I return to the hospital in two weeks. I'm afraid of what they might say. They conduct more exams and review the results. They can't figure it out. "They tell me I'm a mystery," I tell Delia. "Then they take the heart monitor back."

"How does this feel? Do you remember how Lisa feels?"

There's a tug a little higher up in my chest, like a plug is being removed. I take a deep breath. I don't like this feeling. I feel out of control. Tears spill from the corners of my eyes. "I feel empty. Disappointed. I want to know what's wrong with me."

"Lisa, you can ask your body. Your body has an inner physician, and you can ask them questions. Would you like to ask a question?"

"Do you mean aloud?" I ask, mortified.

"If you like. You don't have to. It's your physician. You may talk to them however you like."

As I contemplate this, I start wondering how long I've been here. I try to imagine a little physician inside my body. Then a new image comes to mind. I'm transported back to another nurse's office, but now I'm seven.

I'm visiting the school nurse. I see myself descending a long flight of stairs from my first-grade classroom, holding my hand in agony.

When I get to the nurse's station, the nurse looks at me with concern. "What's wrong?" he asks. He's of medium build and soft-spoken, with a brown beard.

I tell him my finger hurts terribly. He invites me to sit and lays my hand down on the white table. It's cold. He takes out a magnifying glass and asks me how I'm doing. I tell him I've been sleeping on the floor because my baby brother is crying too loudly. He says I look exhausted.

Pointing to a hangnail on my pinky finger, he says, "Aha! This must be the guy!" He takes out clippers and gets to work. I sniffle. It does hurt. When he's finished, he spreads ointment on my pinky and puts on a Band-Aid. He tells me to come back anytime I want to.

Interrupting my daydream, Delia says, "Take your time, Lisa. Your inner physician is always there. You can summon them."

I think again about that summer before college, how worried I was and how I didn't know why. It was the summer before my depression began, before I was hospitalized, before a whole number of terrible violations and humiliations occurred. I wonder, *What was wrong? Was anything really wrong?* I tell Delia about all the questions that weren't asked, like, *How much did I eat? Was I sleeping? How much did I drink? How much did I smoke? Was I lonely? Afraid? Did I have friends?* As I ask these questions, I have an image of my younger self, wearing earphones, blasting music. "I don't think she can hear anything," I say.

"You can ask these questions now," says Delia. "Your body knows."

For as long as I can remember, I've had this feeling that something is terribly wrong with me. I have been searching for answers for as long as I can remember, trying to figure it out. I am always racing from one thing to another. I always feel a sense of tremendous urgency.

"Tell me more about this monitor, Lisa. Where did it go? Is there something wrong with your heart? What does your heart have to say?"

I'm back in the room, a breeze on my face. I shake my head. "I didn't need the monitor. I never needed the monitor."

"What do you need? Does your heart need anything? You can ask."

I feel her closer to my chest. I don't know where her hands are, and I don't want to open my eyes. "What are you doing?"

"I'm loosening the area around your heart. It is still very tight here. Let's listen together."

For what seems like an eternity, she holds her palms over my heart. I feel a flutter and then hear a thumping, like someone knocking, like music. I hear Delia step around the table and stand behind me. She slides her soft, cool hands under my shoulders and lifts my back. I exhale. She slides her hands upward toward my neck and lifts my skull. She turns my head from side to side. It feels like a rush of wind blows through me. It's like there's no gravity. I have no worries. Everything is as it should be. She stands for a few moments, cradling my head like I'm an infant. I let the weight of my head drop more and release the last bits of mental struggle.

"Good work, Lisa. Thank you. Take your time." Delia leaves the room.

When the door closes, I move my palms up to my heart and let them rest there, one on top of the other. I sense a new freedom as I connect with what is already mine. According to yoga philosophy, our greatest intelligence lives in our hearts, not in our minds. Known as "Atman," it refers to the self or the soul. I try to ask my heart the questions that are really plaguing me. *What is wrong with me?* After some time, I ask instead, *Is there something wrong? Can I fix it?* I let my thoughts wander. Eventually a new thought emerges: *What if nothing is wrong?* I ask a follow-up: *What else do I need to know?* I wonder if these mystery symptoms are more like a longing, a longing for myself, for my own presence. This feels true, and I start to envision the heart beneath my hand. *I'm here. I am not going to abandon you. You are a source of direction and truth, and I am responsible for listening to you.* I imagine the hard black plastic monitor from the hospital and make it beautiful, something I can hear, hold, and receive. Instead of a monitor, I imagine my own personal transistor radio, which I can tune into whenever I want. I just need to be patient as I turn the dial past the static, until I find the right station clear as day.

I lie there and listen. The longer I listen, the more I can hear the sounds outside: a bird singing, a horn honking, people laughing. I remember there's a world outside and that I am a part of it. I take a few deep breaths. I don't have any answers to the questions I arrived with, but I have a new radio station, my inner self, and a message I can hear whenever I turn the dial and listen.

On Listening

Kim Thai is an Emmy award–winning producer, writer, social justice advocate, educator, founder of GaneshSpace, and practicing Buddhist in the Thich Nhat Hanh Plum Village tradition.

Listening is probably the most underutilized tool that we have to understand ourselves. Mainly because people's perception of it is that it's so passive. Listening is synonymous with being conscious. Listening is mindfulness; is being awake. Listening is being present, really fully present in what we're doing, and who we're talking to, and what our body is telling us, and absorbing that in a way that doesn't feel overwhelming but provides insight and data to us that is helpful.

Now that your body is awake and we have created space, it's time to relax so you can receive and listen. This is the start of a new regimen that's rooted in science and mindfulness practices that instruct how our listening bodies exist in the world. We'll look both at how we take in stories and what it does to our bodies when we do. This is the toggle and the practice of listening.

The best, most time-honored way to listen is through stillness and relaxation practices. In this section, I'll walk you through a sampling of relaxation exercises, meditations, and breath exercises to strengthen an overall orientation toward stillness. Some may work better for you than others.

Please take care of yourself here. None of these practices is a one-size-fits-all. What feels yummy to some might feel frightening to others. We all take our baggage with us everywhere we go, including when we enter these pages. So please pay attention. If something feels uncomfortable or anxiety-producing in any way, please move away. Skip it. It only takes one practice to sustain you, so if you find one that works, you can stay with it and repeat.

Listening Instinct

Listening is a natural instinct, just like eating, breathing, or expelling. We are all born good listeners, but somewhere along the way, many of us forget or unlearn how to listen. Sometimes it's safer for us emotionally to not really hear everything around us and to close ourselves off. In fact, a recent study showed that in an average conversation, an American adult takes in and comprehends less than 25 percent of what they hear, meaning all of our communication, conversations, texts, and emails are an ongoing game of telephone. We miss the meaning a great portion of the time.

There are very real consequences. When we don't listen to each other, we enter unnecessary conflict, including toxic conversations, fights, and major misunderstandings. We also lose a connection to our own voice and the story we are meant to tell. The good news is listening is teachable and renewable. The best way to practice being heard is to practice listening to another.

Listening is something you are born with, something you have access to and that you can relearn. Before I go any further, let's be clear that the kind of listening I'm talking about has little to do with the ears; the kind of listening I'm talking about is a state of being—of meeting the present moment. What I'm talking about happens with the whole body, in how we pay attention to and communicate with verbal and nonverbal cues. It's a natural biological function.

We see this kind of listening in nature all around us—the way flowers close tight at night, animals freeze in the face of danger, and even how the seasons move between hibernation in the winter to the lush open expanse of summer. Since we are part of nature, we can observe this flow in ourselves as well, in how we listen both to ourselves and to each other. When we are regulated and relaxed, we also have a natural ability to listen, receive, and uncover our authentic voice.

Listening begins with listening to yourself. Listening to the stories your body is holding; the stories your body is cooing, singing, or screaming; and the stories your body is whispering or keeping to itself. Now that you have spent time waking up your stories, you can attune yourself to comprehending those messages; you can begin to move authentically through the world and process your own experiences, making room for listening to others.

Listening and the Nervous System

Listening is a natural extension of our nervous system. When we are stressed, or in fear, we are closed off from our own authentic voice and from others. When we are relaxed, open, and comfortable, we are receptive, and we also digest and release with ease. So in order to listen, we need to take actions to support our own receptivity, and we need to skillfully and mindfully release stories we don't need to make room for new ones. We can think of listening as a state of being that runs parallel to and in sync with a state of rest and restore. Listening and being able to listen is a reliable side effect of being in a relaxed state.

At this point, we're familiar with the idea that our nervous system offers various responses to help us survive and thrive in the outside world. This system works pretty well, but it is *ancient*. We're basically rolling around in vehicles that are thousands of years old and designed to protect us from being chased by lions and that sort of thing. Our systems are not very nuanced and can only shift into one gear at a time—fight, flight, freeze, or fawn, or rest and digest. Fight or flight refers to when we respond to threat by resisting with force or by running away. Freeze is when we put our system on pause or "play dead" to avoid danger; this may emerge in the form of getting very still and being artificially calm or quiet. Fawn is when we respond to a threat by offering people-pleasing behaviors such as flattery. When we stay in one gear too long, we become imbalanced and chock-full of hormones that are harmful in large quantities. This causes a world of problems when our systems are in chronic stress, as most people's are. Since our systems aren't going to get an upgrade anytime soon, at least that I'm aware of, we have to work with what we have. Mindfulness, relaxation, and breath practices give us tools to fine-tune, sensitize, and finesse our operating system and shift from a stress response to rest and digest.

In addition to our nervous system, it's worth noting a couple of other systems that affect our ability to listen, such as our emotional body and our gut sense. Each speaks in a slightly different dialect, protecting us in different ways, to help us understand the world around us. We can think of the gut as our inner GPS or intuition, our general knowledge of whether we feel safe. Our emotional body gives us waves of emotion to instruct our behavior. This is also true on a skeletal and muscular level.

These layers protect us, and they separate us. We've already covered how they protect us, alerting us through feelings and instincts when to be afraid and act. Here's how they separate us: When you're stressed out, afraid, panicking, or disassociating, your body sounds a natural fire alarm in the form of a hormone called cortisol. Cortisol primes you to escape, run, or fight if needed. On a physical level, it makes your muscles contract, your blood thicken, and your breaths become shallow, like you're running. The problem is that if we stay in this state for too long, it runs our system ragged, and we end up suffering from a host of common, problematic, and avoidable diseases, like high blood pressure, diabetes, heart disease, and so on.

Also, problems arise because our ancient system, which isn't very precise, can't discern between a life-threatening stress (like being chased by a bear) and something stressful and annoying (like an email from your boss).

On a listening level, this response is catastrophic. It cuts us off from mindful, whole-body listening and communicating. When you're in this state, it's impossible to receive anything because your body becomes a little Mack truck. Ever try to reason with a Mack truck? When you are in fight or flight, you are primed and designed to identify threats. It is by definition against your nature to rest and restore, befriend, listen, or connect.

Inside, your organs contract and harden to protect themselves from physical harm, which also makes it impossible to receive or digest anything. This is why when you're upset, your stomach aches; or when you're stressed, you can't tap into creative inspiration; or when you're fearful, you can't receive love. When we go into protection mode, we shield ourselves from everything, not just the bad stuff.

The Practice of Listening

The benefits of listening have a potent ripple effect in every area of your creative life. Listening is a way of inviting inspiration and connection and of stoking curiosity in the outside world and in others, encouraging a broader interest in possibilities. In many respects, listening is the home of all creative activity. Listening also provides tangible benefits for a wide range of people. There are ample studies that show that deep listening is restorative for dementia, depression, and anxiety, to name a few. In my experience, one good way to practice listening is through a meditation practice. Meditation itself can be described as a form of listening. Paolo Coelho, author of international bestseller *The Alchemist*, says, "Praying is talking to the Universe. Meditation is listening to it." The two share certain characteristics: a settling and stillness in the body and a capacity to receive or go inward. Many people think they can just come in from their busy day, sit down, and meditate—just like we assume we can toggle between emails and social media while listening to a friend's heartfelt words. When it doesn't work, we're surprised—but we shouldn't be. We do not necessarily arrive in every situation or every day ready to listen. It requires some preparation, just like how meditation requires the stretches and strengthening exercises of yoga poses to ready ourselves to sit and be with our minds. But yoga isn't the only physical practice that supports listening. In fact, all the movement practices described in Part One, and countless other mindful movement forms you may discover on your own, are designed to wake up the body so that it can be at rest.

Listening and Creativity

This stage of pausing, thinking, and waiting for the next thought may also bring about creative impulses. Some of the greatest masterpieces of our time come from this kind of place. Toni Morrison famously shared that she spent three years *thinking* about her award-winning classic *Beloved* before writing a single word. She spent that time listening to what the story had to tell her.

It can also bring about a sense of lasting peace and resilience that you can draw on irrespective of what is going on around you. Herbert Benson, director of the Institute of Mind-Body Medicine at Mass General Hospital, conducted studies on meditators that proved meditation, and restorative yoga, can effectively turn off the stress response—that instinct to close up and freeze in the face of threat, or in our context, when we stop listening—and activate a healing, restorative response. (Read his seminal book *The Relaxation Response* if you're interested in more on that research.) The promise here is powerful; once you learn how to bring yourself into the relaxation response, you'll be able to return to it again and again with greater ease, even in stressful situations. And it's in this relaxed state where we can really listen to each other and connect to a broader humanity outside of ourselves.

When we meditate, we start to pay attention, perhaps for the first time or in a new way. As you listen, you can begin to embody your own healing potential for yourself and for those around you.

In order to awaken our creative impulse, we need to be able to listen to each other and ourselves; this is how we heal. Our healing trajectories and craft excellence run on parallel tracks—in other words, our writing and sharing experience improves as we heal, and we become more self-aware.

Scan Your Body

The only way to know what stories you're carrying is to ask your body.

Listening can be a form of care. It's a way to make space for others and lift their voice. This begins with you. When you listen to all parts of yourself, you offer healing and attention to parts that are ignored. In doing so, you practice doing this for others as individuals and as groups.

A body scan is almost like taking attendance. As you scan your body, explore your inner world and listen to any parts of you that have something to say. As you explore, notice parts that have a lot to say, notice the loud talkers—or even screamers.

Next pay attention to the quieter ones, the ones using inside voices—or even whispering. Pay attention to what they have to say.

Last, and most important, notice if any parts are being quiet.

Ask them what they need; keep them company. Let them know it's okay not to talk. Let them know they're not alone. You are here, listening with love, like a mindful boom operator.

You might want to record yourself reading this aloud and then play it back to practice.

Try it!

Find a comfortable seat or lie down.

Take a few rounds of breath and notice it moving in your body.

Invite your body to relax and bring along an imaginary mic.

Invite your feet to relax; breathe into your heels, soles, toes, and arches. Lift your mic up to your feet and listen to what they might have to say.

Now, move up to your ankles and calves. Breathe in and out like you are fanning a flame. Lift your mic up to your ankles and calves. Listen to what they might have to say.

Now, move up to your legs, knees, and thighs, and let them relax completely. Lift your mic up to your legs, knees, and thighs. Listen to what they might have to say.

Now, let your hips, buttocks, and lower back release into the support beneath you. Lift your mic up to your hips. Listen to what they might have to say.

Let your imagination move up to your torso, lungs, and midback. Breathe and allow your belly to rise and fall. Move the mic around your torso. Listen to what it might have to say.

Now, relax the arms, shoulders, and hands. Let the shoulders relax more. Lift your mic up to your arms and shoulders. What do you hear?

Keep moving until you reach your throat, face, and head. Take a few breaths in and out; relax the jaw and the eyes. Hover the mic over your head. Listen to what it might have to say.

On an in breath, fill the whole body and let go completely. Take a few breaths here.

Repeat the breathing and consider saying silently to yourself, "I have a body. I am enough right in this moment."

Write it!

What did you hear? Who was loud? Who was quiet? Was any part silent?

Listen to Your Ancestors

You carry the voices of your ancestors in your blood and in your bones when you approach the page.

Old stories impact your creative life. They can carry inspiration and guidance. Sometimes their voices encourage and sometimes they hinder. One important thing to remember is you get to decide which ancestors to invite to help guide, protect, and inspire you—and equally important which ancestors to *disinvite*. Your ancestors don't need to be blood relations. They can be important influences and guides both real and imagined. You can listen to them with your body.

As Kim Thai says,

> Listening manifests on a very subconscious physical level in our bodies that we may not even know what the root is because it wasn't in our lifetime. We inherit things we may not even be aware of, that our mothers might not even be aware of. It's less about tracing a sensation back to its origins, but more so being open to the idea that it's more than what I'm experiencing in that moment, that it has more roots beyond what my relationship to it is in that particular moment in time. We can explore listening to our ancestors by investigating, why do I flinch when I hear someone being overly critical of a woman in a space, for example. Or why do I get goosebumps when I hear someone giving an empowering speech? The magic is digging deeper and digging in.

You can ask past generations for guidance. Your ancestors speak to you through your body; they can offer healing direction and inspiration on the page and in your life. In some cases, these guides may appear as much older or younger versions of yourself. They may appear and let you know you're not alone.

Try it!

Take a few rounds of breath and find your seat. As you begin to relax, bring to mind an ancestor you would like to invite into your space. This could be a blood relation; someone you admire, like a writer, teacher, artist, or leader; or someone who has influenced your lineage. Pause and inquire if anyone else is present (sometimes we have other spirits hanging around that we're not even aware of). Now begin a dialogue with them, any kind of dialogue. You can ask them questions, ask for help. You can even offer to help.

The first step is to listen to what they have to say. At first it might feel like a distraction, but then it may free you. Surrender to the stories that need to be told, including the ones you've inherited. You get to choose who you bring with you when you write.

Write it!

Which ancestor is present with you today? Invite them into a conversation. Write down the dialogue.

Quiet Enough to Hear Silence

You must be friends with silence to hear.
—Joy Harjo, poet laureate of the United States, 2019–2022[8]

Under certain conditions silence can be a gateway to universal magic, truth, and creative flow. Silence can offer an invitation to something unknown, something mysterious and connected to a greater spiritual realm. However, it's not always so simple to find it or feel comfortable there.

Silence can also be threatening. It can come in the form of oppression and repression, in the silencing and erasing of vulnerable stories; it can come in the form of silence or apathy from a bystander who doesn't use their voice. In many settings, if it's *too* quiet, it can also mean danger is lurking. Perhaps the most powerful obstacle to finding serenity in silence lies within each of us: our own minds get very noisy, distracted, and even distressed when we get quiet.

Befriending silence is personal and requires getting to know it. How can you be quiet enough to make room for the voice within?

Write it!

Approach silence like it is a friend. Personify the silence you're waiting for. What are they like?

On the Concept
of Creating Silent Space

Jessica Kung Dreyfus is the founder of Make Conscious and explores the concept of creating silent space.

If you're silent but your mind is racing, you're not silent. You need to get to a place of some relative stillness. When you put your mind on an object, it doesn't necessarily stay on that object. The normal consciousness of our world is the mind bounces from one object to another. So, let's say you don't meditate, but you shut yourself in your room, like in COVID quarantine; you may even not talk, but there's no silence. There's still noise and business. Before you even close your eyes, you need to stop and see and calibrate your mind stuff. Silence is one of the ways you start to see the true nature of the mind, which for most of us is pretty cluttered. The pace of our life is such that there is no space for stillness.

Silence helps you navigate that liminal space and allows you to navigate your mind.

Jessica offers the following suggestion for finding silence:

I think an hour is a great start. For me it just starts by creating a space in your house to even have the hour. People get pulled out of their hour by their TV, by their phone. Before you even start the hour, you literally need to unplug everything that beeps, that takes your attention, that beeps or buzzes. Maybe your home isn't the place. If you're at home, you literally need to airplane mode everything. Then create that container and do whatever you want to do in that hour. You can read, write, draw and do whatever you want. But you need to create that non interruption, or otherwise the phone will ring, your doorman will buzz. It just takes an instant to take you out of the silence because your mind is not used to it. We're used to just pressing a button.

Listening Medicine

Hearing and telling stories are integral to healing. When hearing stories about healing from people who seem like us, we become inspired to believe that our own healing is possible.
—Dr. Lewis Mehl Madrona, integrative healer and author of *Narrative Medicine*[9]

I think most people know it's important to listen on some level, but maybe we'd take more actions to protect this valuable resource if we understood its power a bit more. Hearing stories is integral to our healing and sense of belonging. Listening is one of our most powerful resources, yet in our medical system, the average doctor has less than eighteen minutes to spend with each patient. Our most important caregivers are operating under incredible strain, time scarcity, and mountains of paperwork. Their nervous systems barely stand a chance at setting up their bodies to listen, care, and diagnose effectively.

Beyond the accuracy of a diagnosis, it's in the hearing of our own stories inside and outside of the medical establishment that accelerates our own healing trajectory. On a societal, medical, interpersonal, and political level, the implications are huge. We're living in a time defined by apartness, difficulty, disease, and distress. We harm each other on a daily basis in micro-nonlistening moments. Making changes to the way we listen, both to ourselves and to those around us, can radically alter our sense of wellness and lived experience.

Contemplate it!

How can you protect listening space? How can you make more time to listen?

Listening Is Radical

Receiving something we don't already know is the risk—and reward—we get by listening.

Another way of understanding listening is as the process of leaving your interior thoughts and opening yourself up to the world with all its suffering and chaos, alongside all its joy and love. These messages are not always spoken, or even written; they're communicated in our bodies' vibrations, sounds, and movements. Receiving this kind of information might be scary to imagine, which is why we might avoid true listening in our daily lives. We can't always prepare for what we'll hear with our bodies, making listening an act of radical faith— in ourselves and the world we're a part of. We need to be willing to receive something unknown.

Entering willingly into listening is easier when we feel physically grounded, which provides a foundation of trust, healing, and compassion. Legendary listener and founder of the On Being Project, Krista Tippet, talks about listening as "present awareness" and "wonderment." She writes, "Generous listening is powered by curiosity, a virtue we can invite and nurture in ourselves to render it instinctive. It involves a kind of vulnerability—a willingness to be surprised, to let go of assumptions and take in ambiguity."[10]

Opening ourselves to be changed by what we hear does much more than change our individual lives.

Contemplate it!

Pause to acknowledge how much courage it takes to do what you are doing right now.

Honor Changes and Cycles

Observing natural cycles is a way of listening to the world around us as it is.

We are part of the natural world, and as such we are always moving through changes and cycles—whether we are circling the sun and hitting another birthday or major milestone or noticing the seasons outside of us or within us. We're affected by changes, challenges, hormonal shifts, aging. Gracefully accepting and moving with these cycles is a way of addressing our basic wellness and well-being. Sometimes simply naming them, becoming aware that they exist, places them in proper alignment.

Write it!

Name any cycle you are aware of that is impacting you.

How is it affecting you? Is there a clear beginning, middle, and end?

Find Calm in the World

Sit upright but not uptight.

When I first walked through the doors of a meditation center in my neighborhood about a decade ago, I felt desperate, like I was skating across the bottom of life. All the tools I had to help me manage states of anxious depression, apartness, and hyperarousal had ceased working. I felt so uncomfortable in my skin that I was willing to try anything. I noticed that people who meditated seemed to be calmer, more comfortable, and even happier. I wanted that and had a knowing sense that if I surrounded myself with folks like this, it might rub off on me. I scoured the area and chose a spot where my dear friend Ethan Nichtern taught.

When I arrived at the studio, the last thing in the world I wanted to do was sit still. But I mirrored the others in the room, finding a few cushions to stack on top of each other and taking a seat. The idea of sitting in a room with my eyes closed surrounded by strangers, many of them men, was about as comfortable as taking a bath in boiling water, in public. Imagine my relief when Ethan said the method he would be teaching involved keeping the eyes open and setting a relaxed gaze. He described that the idea behind this practice was that we were in training to be awake in the world. He referred to this as "being a warrior in the world." I sure *thought* I knew how to be a warrior. Then he instructed us to "sit upright but not uptight." I began to find ease.

In his seminal book *The Road Home*, he writes, "Eventually, if we are going to wake up and truly come home to our own heartmind, we have to turn the full scope of our life into a practice space. This doesn't have to start as an all-the-time endeavor, but little by little it is said that our awareness practice can become a constant companion."[11]

I returned to the center and studied for some time, and as time went on, I found a lot of comfort in keeping my eyes open. I began a personal practice at home. Practicing meditation like this, or another form you choose, consistently, over a long period of time, promises to awaken a reflex of finding calm awareness no matter what is going on. For lots of emotional and practical reasons, it's not always possible or comfortable to close your eyes. You don't have to; you can meditate with your eyes open. This open-eyed meditation practice helps you develop a habit of being able to find concentration and calm amid the chaotic world and not be afraid of where or who you are.

You can do this too.

Try it!

1. Find a comfortable seat and become aware of your breath.
2. Set your gaze on the ground about four to six feet in front of you.
3. Focus on an area about a foot wide, not a pinprick. This could also be the glow from a candle or some other object of meaning.
4. Breathe and keep your loose gaze on this general area.
5. As your thoughts wander, bring your mind back to the focal point to help focus your mind and calm your thinking.
6. Try this at first for three minutes; then experiment moving up to five minutes, then ten, and possibly twenty.

When your time is up, allow the breath to grow stronger.

Take any micromovements that are calling to you. Begin to let the gaze lift, and look around the room. Stretch and move in whatever manner you like.

Write it!

What came up for you during the meditation? What did it feel like? What did you see? What did you think about? Write about a time your attention was pulled away. What brought you back?

Follow the Feeling to the Meaning

Emotions create stories in our bodies for us to understand, express, and share.

Every emotion has a natural wavelength—a beginning, middle, and end. And every emotion has an inherent wisdom and message. Emotions exist to direct our actions. For example, anger can inspire action, sadness can inspire slowing down, happiness can inspire connection, and so on. But we're often cutting them short and losing meaning in the process.

Most of the time, we can't fully access our feelings. We *fine* our way out of our feelings. (How are you doing? *Fine!* I'm fine!) Denying our emotions is a little bit like driving around in a car and deciding not to use the lights, the signals, the mirrors, or the speedometer. Our feelings exist to signal how the outside world is impacting us so we can make the most beneficial decisions on how to behave with ourselves, with each other, and on the page. We need our emotions to survive and to express the beautiful range of our creative visions.

In the same way we needed to wake up our stories, now we need to wake up our feelings. Listening to them is an invitation. Invite them. Name them. Allow them.

Try it!

Find a comfortable seat and take a few rounds of breath to settle. As you settle in, begin to focus on any emotion that is present; this could be joy, anger, sadness, grief, excitement, or something else.

Name one at a time, and stay with them.

Be curious about what it feels like: Do they have a shape or texture? What are any defining features? Stay with each for about five breaths and then move on to a different emotion. Stay with this practice until you have spent time with every feeling you can discover.

Try this practice and be open. You don't need to do anything with this or tell a story about it. Just bear witness and welcome.

Sound Meditation

Silence isn't the absence of sound; it is the absence of noise.

One way to find silence is to listen for it. So, right now, stop what you're doing and listen. What noises are around you? Can you discern the difference between sound and noise?

This practice offers a way to use different sounds as tools to focus and discern and find peace. You can practice this anywhere—in a library or in the middle of Times Square.

Try it!

Find a comfortable seat and take a few rounds of breath.

Locate a sound that feels far away. This might mean outside your window or in a different room. Its source should be out of reach and out of sight. There may be a few sounds competing for your attention. Take a few moments to choose one that will hold your interest. Stay with that sound for one minute. If your mind wanders to another sound or idea, allow it, and then, on an in breath, return to your faraway sound.

Now choose a sound that is nearby. This could even be a sound you are making, like your breath or your heartbeat. Stay with that sound. Again, if your mind wanders, return to that sound. It's okay. Your mind will wander. On an in breath, bring it back to the nearby sound and stay with it. Stay with this sound for one minute.

Next, let go of that and bring your attention to the sensation of your breath moving in your body. Stay with this sensation for at least one minute.

Modification

Try this with a vibration or sensation that feels far away and a vibration or sensation that feels close.

Write it!

Describe what you heard. Did you notice any sensations in your body? Did any memories come up? Did you prefer one sound over another?

Rest and Digest Stories

Once you have processed information properly, you'll have space to take in new stories and be present with your own.

We often think about digestion relating to the foods and liquids we consume, but we also consume measurable amounts of electronic, audio, emotional, and visual information throughout the day that we need to process and digest. Digestion is another way to describe listening. We feel the impact of what we consume through our ears almost immediately and all over the body: in our gut, our back, our head, our heart. When we're stuffed to the gills, it's impossible to process information or take in anything new.

This gentle twist supports digestion in several ways. It gently rings out the intestines, encouraging smooth processing of food. It also releases tension in the belly, the lower back, and all the way up the spine to the neck, helping the body, mind, and spirit move into a more relaxed state. So it's a good practice for physical digestion, but it's also good if you had a big "meal" of information that's not sitting well with you.

This can be done on the ground before bed or first thing in the morning.

Try it!

Lying down:
Lie down on a padded surface, like a mat or even a bed.
Turn yourself over to your side, bending your knees. Bend your elbow and lift your head onto the support of your palm (otherwise known as "lying on the beach" pose).

Bend the top leg, drape it over a pillow or folded blanket, and
lengthen the lower leg.

Relax into the support that's already there and breathe into your
lower gut, relaxing and releasing. Ideally, stay here for twenty
minutes, allowing any difficult conversations or pieces of
information or news to arise on an in breath and release on
an out breath.

Seated:

Sit on the edge of your seat, and plant your feet on the ground a
little wider than hip-distance apart.

Inhale and reach your hands out, around, and up to frame above
your head.

Twist to the right. Let your right hand rest on the arm or back of
the chair and your left hand rest on your thigh.

Breathe into this twist for three rounds of breath.

Inhale to an upright position and repeat on the other side.

Write it!

What do you need help digesting? Is it something you read, heard,
or experienced? Is it a feeling or a memory?

Change the Way You Listen by Changing What You Say

Expand your heart as you work with difficult experiences, thoughts, and people.

When we adopt the writing body posture—the rounded spine, downward gaze, curved and isolated shape—our thoughts, opinions, and judgments move in that direction too. Judgment, suspicion, and detachment can be a natural effect of how we live. It takes constant and consistent effort to shift a worldview toward openness, connection, and trust. We have tried some physical postures and breath exercises; this meditation practice is another option.

This ancient practice, called Metta meditation or loving-kindness meditation, was taught by the Buddha thousands of years ago. Beloved meditation teacher and pioneer Sharon Salzberg studied this technique in Burma in the 1980s and brought these teachings back to the United States; since then, she has been inspiring millions across the globe through her books, teachings, and talks.

This practice is an ancient framework to rest our attention on the silent repetition of a version of these four phrases: May you be safe. May you be happy. May you be healthy. May you have ease. The repetition of these words serves as a conduit for paying attention; these repeated phrases expand your worldview because you don't stop with yourself but move on to other people—those you know and those you don't. Ultimately, this practice encourages an experience of interconnectedness. Over time you can experience an embodied feeling of what this is like. Salzberg writes, "Metta is the ability to embrace all parts of ourselves, as well as all parts of the world. Practicing Metta illuminates our inner integrity because it relieves us of the need to deny different aspects of ourselves. We can open to everything with the healing force of love."[12]

Try it!

The goal of Metta is to cultivate loving-kindness toward all beings, including yourself. It's also been proven to reduce negative emotions, decrease anxiety, and enhance personal connections and self-love.

To begin, find a seat and take a few breaths.

Personalize these four statements:

1. May you be safe.
2. May you be happy.
3. May you be healthy.
4. May you have ease.

Next, think of a beloved, someone or something in your life who is really easy to love, and apply those statements. Spend a minute repeating, "May [their name] be safe, may they be happy, may they be healthy, may they have ease." Keep your attention on one statement at a time; try not to skip ahead.

Next, think of a familiar stranger, someone you see but don't know well, such as a barista or neighbor. Spend a minute repeating, "May [their image] be safe, may they be happy, may they be healthy, may they have ease."

Next, think of a difficult person, someone who is annoying you, and spend a minute repeating, "May [their name] be safe, may they be happy, may they be healthy, may they have ease."

Finally, think of yourself. It might be useful to imagine a familiar photo of yourself from childhood. Then spend a minute repeating, "May I be safe, may I be happy, may I be healthy, may I have ease."

You can do this all day long.

Reading Is Listening Too

Find an increased feeling of integration and balance.

When you read on a screen or a printed page, as you read your eyes are moving back and forth, from left to right, in bilateral movements. This back-and-forth is reminiscent of a psychological treatment called eye movement desensitization and reprocessing (EMDR) therapy, which has been proven to have a soothing effect on the brain as it integrates the left and right brain to help people recover from trauma and difficult emotional experiences.

You don't need to do anything with it; just absorb the fact that reading is soothing on a brain level.

Try it!

Schedule time for reading a few times a week. You can read anything: poetry, a novel, a magazine, a newspaper.

Write it!

Keep a journal about how reading impacts your thinking, moods, and sense of contentment.

Be the Beach

Do nothing. Let others be the waves. Let them
come to you.

Doing nothing can feel like refraining from doing the thing we want
to do or say, but nature offers us another way to think about it. Imagine being more like a beach.

The beach doesn't go leaping out to grab the waves; the beach
stays still and allows the water to come to it. Embody this image
next time you're listening to someone, doing nothing, saying nothing. Simply receiving is some of the most powerful love and healing
we can offer someone else.

A natural outcome of quieting yourself for listening is that you
notice other people's stories, truths, and offerings coming to you
more often. This can be relaxing and rejuvenating for you too. Imagine the beach on a sweet summer day, the waves lapping in.

When you stop trying to control, you can receive intuitive
direction.

Try it!

This one will take a partner. It can be someone in your home or a
friend on the phone. Have a conversation with this person and just
allow them to speak. Do not interrupt them, try to fix anything, or
encourage. Don't exaggerate, exasperate, or inquire. Just listen. Be
the beach. When they seem like they have completed a thought, you
can simply ask, "Is that all? Do you have anything to add?" Thank
them.

Compassion Overload

Pain is inevitable, but suffering is avoidable.

We live in a time when painful stories are all around us—whether it's a war halfway around the world, a client sharing, a neighbor whose mom just died, or a memory within us. No matter the situation, we can get overwhelmed by listening to painful stories. Even professional listeners, like therapists and clergy, doctors and healers, suffer from overload. Thinking about others can prevent you from hearing yourself. Worry, concern, fear, and compassion overload can be the greatest writer's block for many caregiving types.

The solution to this, as with so many solutions in this book, is to allow it, go right toward it, and practice *with* it.

Inspired by a powerful ancient Tibetan Buddhist practice, Tonglen offers a practical framework for managing, flushing, and processing overwhelming stories. Pema Chodron writes, "Tonglen means 'taking in and sending out.' This meditation practice is designed to help ordinary people like ourselves connect with the openness and softness of our hearts. Instead of shielding and protecting our soft spot, with tonglen we could let ourselves feel what it is to be human."[13]

It works to get you out of self and out of worry. It will increase compassion for others and then, as a result, help foster self-compassion and self-love. This can be done for someone you know who is sick and suffering. You can also do this on the spot at a red light when you're driving or at your workplace—anywhere at all where you interact with people.

Find a comfortable seat and soft point of focus for your gaze, like a candle, object of meaning, or a neutral area on the floor.

Begin the visualization by imagining breathing in fire and breathing out cool water. Do this for a few rounds.

Focus on a situation that is real to you—a particular person, place, or entity that is experiencing pain and suffering.

Breathe in their pain or suffering.

Breathe out whatever will benefit them.

Breathe in their pain, suffering, illness, or anguish.

Breathe out love and understanding.

Continue in this way.

After a few minutes, you may expand the visualization so you are no longer focusing only on this one person with this condition but every person with this condition—every person who is suffering. This can include you.

Breathe in pain and breathe out love and compassion for all.

Write it!

Write about the situation that came to mind. What did you breathe in? What did you breathe out?

Soften

A soft heart is the gateway to compassion.

We carry our stories around with us everywhere we go, and sometimes they get heavy. Remember, it's always an option to let go. And it's always an option to let go more. This restorative heart-opening posture supports relaxation and provides an opportunity to shift perspective. Let go and let something new in.

There are a few ways to move into this posture. I'll walk you through a general setup, but please do whatever feels right to you. Our lower body—our hips, legs, and feet—is often associated with emotions, ancestors, family, and challenge.

It will be helpful to have two pillows and a blanket or towel.

Try it!

Lie down, bend your knees, place your feet on the floor, and let your legs fall away to either side while keeping your feet together. You can place pillows under your thighs and your head. Let your legs and feet relax on the floor.

Bring your awareness to your heart, and direct your breath to your heart center.

Take some time to breathe in and out through your heart (anywhere from five to twenty minutes).

Write it!

What does your heart have to say?

On When Does a Sound
Stop Being a Sound?

Sadie Brightman is an acclaimed musician and the founder and executive director of Middlebury Music Center.

As I listened to the tone, it pulled me in. It wasn't a one-to-one ratio with the key. You press the key once, but the sound that is produced is never just one thing. Rather, the tone is in a continuous state of change, it is impermanent. I found that variability to be wildly reassuring. I could interact with its changing nature just by being there, being present, listening. I didn't realize at the time that all the dynamism I heard in the fading tone was also within me. The tone of the key was like a mirror to a vast curiosity inside me, a reserve of inner resources.

As writers, we do this all the time when we're listening for the authentic voice. Whether you're tapping on a keyboard or writing with a pen or dictating, every word, every idea, is like a note. How can you listen to it until it reaches the end?

Write it!

If your story were a note, what would it sound like?

Listen for Oneness

When you learn to listen to a single sound, you can hear the entire universe.

In the middle of my five-hundred-hour yoga training, my teacher, Julie Mellk, stopped class and asked us to sit down and listen. It was a strange thing to do. We were in the middle of a vigorous sequence and many hours into a long day. But we all stopped, sat down, and listened. The studio was located on the second floor of a small building in Soho, in downtown Manhattan. I heard car horns, a hot dog vendor yelling orders, an ambulance siren.

A few moments passed. Julie followed up with, "Do you hear it?" I had no idea what she was talking about and squeezed my face trying to pick up on more. She smiled again at me, "You don't need to try so hard, Lisa. It's all around you, the sound, the sound of om is always there." I sat still, and she repeated, "Do you hear it now?" She added, "Om is widely understood as the vibrational sound of the universe, the vibration from where all vibrations are born."

I didn't hear anything, but I nodded anyway, if only so this awkward moment would pass. It took some time, but as the day wore on, I came to experience how the sounds were melding into one greater sound, one sound, like when you squint and look off into the horizon and everything becomes a blur. The honks and sirens merged with the woman's voice and the breath of the students around me. The sound became one blurry wave. It was beautiful, and I was a part of it.

Through the melding vibrations, I began to feel how interconnected we all are. I started to understand in a sense how sounds—from voices, trucks, cars, airplanes, music, trees, and everywhere else—were coming from and rushing toward the same source. I don't always hear it, but I always know this connecting universal sound is there.

At a certain point, repeated sounds start to come together, and it's hard to discern when one part begins and ends. This is a way of training the ear to listen for unity and interconnectivity—in other words, to listen for what connects us.

You can feel the universal sound wherever you are too.

Try it right now.

Quiet Wildness

To listen is to offer yourself freely to the wild world.

A funny thing happens when you take a walk in the woods seeking quiet: the quieter you get, the louder the natural world becomes. With each step, the crackling of branches beneath your feet, the call of a bird, and the rustling of the wind become more prominent. Our minds are the same way.

Our inner voices speak to us in hushed tones. We can only hear them if we are still and quiet. They're always there to guide us. All we need to do is show up and wait. Sociologist and activist Parker Palmer writes that our spirit is "like a wild animal" and that if you "wish to see a wild animal in the woods the last thing you should do is go crashing about, instead sit quietly and await the wildness you seek."[14]

We've established by now that listening is more than simply being quiet. It's more than focusing on sound coming through your ears. Listening can be thought of as an embodied state of awareness, something that happens with the whole body when we are present. When we can find this place, we can connect with our true vision, our true voice, and we have the potential to reach others as well.

Write it!

What wildness do you seek?

PART THREE

Express

SIX LITTLE LETTERS: *W R I T E R*

I am sitting, uncomfortably, on a yoga mat, notebook in hand, amid about one hundred earnest strangers wrapped in blankets at Dani Shapiro's meditation and writing workshop. It seems everyone but me has created a personal little island comprised of cushions, bolsters, and blocks, like a scene from a giant sleepover—but not like any sleepover I had ever been to. I feel both like I am exactly where I need to be and totally out of my element.

At a certain point, Dani looks out at the group and says, "Raise your hand if you're a writer."

Not a single person raises their hand. I can feel the tension knock against the piles of yoga props. She waits, unflustered by the lack of response. I tentatively glance around and notice a few others doing the same. Like prairie dogs, our heads bop up and down, checking to see if anyone else is going to raise their hand. I start making a mental list, weighing whether I can pass for a *writer*. Sure, I have always kept a journal, and I have published a few articles. I certainly have never published a book, though. I give myself a solid *maybe*. I raise my hand about shoulder level—a kind of half raise to avoid being interpreted clearly either way.

Dani waits a little longer and then offers a warm smile and more formal welcome to the start of the retreat. She gently reminds us we had all set aside this valuable time to pursue writing, to deepen our path. She suggests that we are, in fact, all writers. I feel like a jerk—why didn't I raise my hand? I am desperate to prioritize my writing, to dive deeper into myself and seek meaning. Why can't I put a name on it? As my mind burrows into this questioning, there's a collective release around the room. Why do we all feel unworthy of this title, these six letters: $WRITER$? Why did I feel unworthy?

Writing, a Narrative Healing Practice

Most writing classes jump right in and start writing. What happens is that only the loudest or bossiest story gets told. So many of us are walking around with quieter and sometimes silent stories. Because we spent time allowing the stories in our bodies to open up and wake up and then feel safe and heard, they can now express themselves.

The intention is for this writing practice to be private. It can be quiet, humble, and personal; it can be raw, loud, colorful. It can express the full range of emotions and experiences without any fear of judgment. It's the practice you do with the doors closed, or figuratively or literally out in the wilderness with nobody around but you and your spirit guides and animal friends, a fearless draft that never needs to be read or seen.

This kind of writing is done for the sole purpose of self-reflection; it's a mindfulness practice. It has a lot of names—free writing, journaling, expressive writing—and hundreds of studies have shown that when done under certain conditions, over a period of time, it can have measurable positive effects on your physical and emotional health and sense of overall well-being, including healing from trauma. There are so many benefits to a writing practice, such as improved immune function; lower blood pressure; healing from trauma; reduced stress, anxiety, and depression; increased resilience, sense of connection and belonging, joy, and contentment; and improved sleep, focus, and clarity. Essentially, writing, like yoga, meditation, or any kind of mindful movement (even Olympic weightlifting), can be healing when done consistently over time in earnest effort. It can lead to tremendous results, inspiration, personal transformation, community care, and creative fulfillment—whether you consider yourself a writer or not.

Writing itself is a mindful movement, in a sense. As I mentioned earlier, the back-and-forth motions when our eyes move across the page or across the screen, the back-and-forth motion of the pen, and typing on a keyboard are forms of bilateral motion, which itself is a form of therapy that integrates the brain's two hemispheres and can be key to emotional processing and produce an overall soothing effect on the body.

In this context, writing can be something you add to support an existing self-care practice. If you happen to be a professional writer or creator working on something larger, these practices can act as a spark or fuel. Bottom line: writing can amplify whatever journey you are on. It doesn't need to replace anything you're already doing. It is another tool in your tool kit of healing. If you are working on a creative project, these generative prompts are designed to shake up old stories and ignite your true voice so the story you are meant to share may emerge.

Self-Care and Writing About Trauma

We are all holding trauma stories on some level, whether we experienced a traumatic event personally—or our ancestors did, or a loved one, or we watched something on television. No matter what experience overwhelms your body, writing can be invaluable to you as you approach tender or challenging stories within you or with folks you come into contact with. If you're working with trauma, challenging experiences, or difficult emotions, this practice can be particularly healing for you when done under certain conditions. (We'll talk more about this later.)

You don't need to share anything you write, and if you do, it's highly recommended you work with a trained professional, support group, or specialist when you are writing about trauma to ensure safety and optimal results. I want to underscore it's not always beneficial to share this tender work, and you need to find the right person to listen (more on that in the next part).

I also want to emphasize that you do not need to write about your trauma in order to receive the healing benefits. The act of writing is healing, irrespective of the content. There's been wonderful research done by institutions such as Mass General and Sloan Kettering that prove that patients, even those living with terminal illnesses and grave traumatic experiences, receive measurable benefits from writing—about anything at all! Judith Kelman, founder of Visible Ink, a program for patients at Memorial Sloan Kettering Cancer Center, writes, "Patients encouraged to express themselves creatively feel more in control, less stressed and anxious, and better able to deal with the rigors of treatment."

You may choose to write about something hard, but you don't have to. You can write a poem, a screenplay, a crime novel. All writing can be healing writing. In the back of the book, I will also include some more resources relating to writing and trauma.

On the Concept of Narrative Therapy

Sarah Mandel is a clinical psychologist in New York City and the author of the memoir *Little Earthquakes.*

Writing helped me emerge out of my trauma-induced, dissociated state—which for me included staring at the ceiling, motionless, for hours on end. Even though I was declared alive, I felt dead inside. And I feared that I would always feel that way. Once the clinical psychologist in me realized that I was traumatized, I thought, I wonder if the trauma narrative therapy that I've provided for my patients could help me heal. So I embarked on the treatment for myself, with my personal therapist at the ready if I needed support along my writing path.

Narrative therapy typically entails the writing or re-telling of your trauma in detail. At first, the memories may resemble puzzle pieces in a chaotic heap; but slowly you start to sort them. Over time, you assemble the memories to create a whole story with a beginning, middle, and end.

Interacting with my memories helped me gain a sense of control, which was a profound shift from my previous state of helplessness. We often attempt to push memories away or try to stop emotions from bubbling up, but our brains simply don't know how to avoid our internal experience. In order to heal, we need to feel everything and let the pain be released out of our minds and bodies. The form of expression can vary, and include writing, oral re-telling, painting, something to bring the traumatic experience out into the light of day, to look at it in the safety of the present. You learn that what you went through was real, and you accept that your reactions, though seemingly bizarre, actually make sense given your terrifying ordeal. Once you complete your narrative it becomes clear that your trauma is in the past, and there is hope for the future.

Set an Intention

Writing is like yoga, or meditation, or playing the piano, gardening, or really any other practice; you enjoy it more and receive more benefits the more you do it. This is one way of thinking about what it means to create an intention. Setting an intention before you do something magnifies its impact and your likelihood of success.

Another, more spiritual way to think about this is that setting an intention creates a seal around your practice and separates the work from the grind of daily life.

Let's take a moment to pause and set an intention for today's practice.

Take a new breath and listen for guidance and direction. What brings you here today? Do you have a purpose or goal? Is there a story you're ready to share? Is there something you want to achieve or learn? Are you growing? Is there someone you would like to devote your practice to? Focus on something within reach, something you can almost smell and taste.

Write it!

Write your intention.

Go Where You Feel Good

If you remember it, you can return to it.

It's an unremarkable Monday morning, and every eye in the room is glued to the clock as if it is about to come alive. No one is listening to a word Mr. Hubner, our English teacher, is saying. After some time passes, he slams his notebook closed and says, "Okay, that's it! Everyone, take out your notebooks and pens. For the remainder of class, I want each of you to write about wherever you wish you were right now."

We are rapt. Pens fly across the page. For the next thirty minutes, the only sound is the scratch of pen on paper, and the occasional sigh. The room is humming with creativity.

I write about the feeling of sun on my skin, lying on a smooth rock on an island in the middle of the Atlantic Ocean next to my friend Susan. It is a remarkable moment. Instead of eighteen grumpy adolescents sitting in a circle at cold hard desks, we are transported to the places we love most. Afterward, to our horror, he asks us to go around the room and share what we wrote.

Ethan writes about a memory of being in the supermarket with his mom. Molly tells a story about hiking. Someone else writes about their bed. As we share, we hover in a new space of connection and shared memories and friendship.

Taking yourself to a place that brings comfort and ease in your mind is the concept of "remembered wellness," a phrase coined by Herbert Benson, whom I mentioned earlier. He suggests that it could arise in meditation and stillness practices, like restorative yoga, but we can also find this feeling through our creative practice by deeply listening to where our hearts want to take us. Looking back, I can see how this prompt relaxed our nervous systems and transformed our impatient, sullen bodies into bodies full of connection and warmth and willingness.

Once you find this place, you can carry it with you no matter what the circumstances outside are. You will be able to summon your truth and be present with what is. This is how you find your home base in real time.

Now it's your turn.

Write it!

Where do you wish you were right now?

What Keeps You from Writing Your Story?

You can express who you truly are.

We all have inner critics and obstacles that prevent us from sharing our truth. We think we're protecting ourselves by telling them to be quiet. *You better not say that. Don't you dare. Be careful.* Eventually, we let them speak to us in our own voice. These obstacles can also stem from critical feedback from dominant culture and the outside world.

As Kim Thai says,

> Often dominant culture wants to make us smaller, wants us to have one story, which right now is cis white skinny and able bodied and hetero. The work here is how do you relate to this story, and do you question your worthiness. How can you identify that that is just a story, and you can either give power to it or let it go with lots and lots of internal work of excavating that out. And how can you express yourself in a way that truly claims you as you truly are. All these stories carry so much power because they police us, they disempower us, they harm us. The more we can use discernment, the more we can filter out what doesn't work for us.

Write it!

Bring to mind anything or anyone that blocks you, criticizes you, judges you, or makes you feel limited or oppressed. Is it a person? Someone who criticizes or devalues you? Or a system? An experience?

What would you write if that thing, or place, or system weren't there?

On How We Tell Stories
with Our Bodies

Eva Ludwig is a trauma therapist, yoga teacher, and somatic therapist.

Biases are just the stories that we tell ourselves and the stories we hold about others. That can be about power, about any area of oppression whatsoever. Just like any story or memory or experience that gets stored in our brain and our bodies, those stories about power differentials are also stored in our bodies. Storytelling is the ultimate disrupter. When we're able to bring ourselves into it and notice what's going on in ourselves, we're able to release that.

You don't need to know the solution or how to fix racism or fix sexism or fix the fact that women's rights are being dismantled by our government. It's about noticing that something is happening in your body. That's what lets me know that something is off, and I wonder what that's about. It gives us a way to be curious and a way in so that we can then communicate.

Eyes on Your Page

Keep the focus on you.

Writing begins as an inward-facing art. When we sit down to work and only think of what others will think, we're guaranteed to get stuck.

In my years working with writers, one of the most common obstacles I have witnessed is an excessive preoccupation with others. Others can mean your reader, reviewer, editor, family member. It can mean your sixth-grade English teacher or even something more amorphous, like your own private bogeyman or monster.

Here's one thing I've also noticed about writers who pledge their allegiance to their critic: getting stuck doesn't necessarily mean you won't write. You may write a lot. In fact, I've worked with several writers who wrote whole series of books in service of these critics, but what they all have in common is a deep dissatisfaction with the work itself.

Writing from the outside in means you may not write the true story that your body, right now, needs you to share. It is possible to live with and beyond the critic, or monster, or trauma, or obstacle that will arise as you write. Embrace them. One solution is to befriend this critic, and the fastest way to befriend is to listen.

Write it!

Write an ode to your critic.

Writing Space

The only way to design the space of our inner
lives is through practice and designing a
practice that works.

We go nuts planning the perfect place to write. We buy the perfect
incense and candles. We surround ourselves with the right lighting,
music, paintings, books, colors. We write from our bedrooms, cars,
studios, cafés. But the only space we can really control is within.

Write it!

Describe your writing practice as it actually is. (This might include
something like, *I do not currently have a writing practice.*) Keep going.

Establish a Routine

There are so many myths about what it takes to be a writer. The most important thing is to find a routine that works for you.

I've worked with writers who work every day at 5:00 a.m. and others who only write at night. I knew a best-selling author who *only* wrote on Wednesday evenings. I have another friend who only writes on Saturdays.

Some of the happiest and most productive people I know do the same thing every day. They live lives defined by simple routines and rituals. This is the bedrock of most spiritual practices around the globe, where the community follows set times for prayer, meditation, eating, movement, creativity, and service. These routines act like an inspiration container.

Scan the week you just experienced. Recall when and where you had natural pockets of time to write (or spend the next week observing this). Build a schedule around what works for you and your life as it actually is. Consider the conditions you need, where and when you might find privacy. Put your phone on "do not disturb."

Write it!

What are the routines in your life that support your self-care and creativity? Write about them. Be specific and realistic. Keep in mind the following:

Time of day
Place
Length of practice
Other obligations
Rituals for beginning or ending
What else?

Writing Blocks Are Gifts and Opportunities

But as writers, we should use everything that touches us. It's all ore to be refined into story.

—Octavia Butler[15]

Try to recall a time when you didn't know the next step or what to do next, where to turn or what to say, and then, out of nowhere, you had a new thought. What guided you back to the path, even if it was a different one than where you started? When we check in with our inner guide, there is a power at work that's hard to put into words. Some call it energy, force, or spirit; you could call it intuition, inspiration, instinct, muse, or God. Whatever you call it, it works on a different sphere from the verbalized world in which we live most of the time. It's a feeling of connection, being supported, guided, and inspired. It's something you can always trust, call on, and rely on.

Write it!

Describe a time you felt blocked and then found your way out. What happened?

Keep Moving

As you write, you let go of what holds you back.

There's a traditional Chinese medicine practice to energetically "cut" the cords to free yourself so you can have a new experience. Free writing is something like that.

Put the pen to paper and spend the next ten minutes writing down anything that comes to mind. Even if you're just writing *I have nothing to say*. The idea is to put the pen to paper and allow it to keep moving. Cut the cord from whatever it is you think you should say.

Write it!

Free write for fifteen minutes. Write whatever comes to mind and keep going.

Design a Moat

There is an energy within you that is healing, limitless, abundant—and it is just for you.

Too often we dole out our precious energy to other people and petty distractions. We all know what happens right after we dream up the perfect space: *something* happens to distract us. Maybe you need to make a dentist appointment; or your partner is sick; or your kid, boss, friend, or neighbor needs something, everything, from you. The list can be endless.

In her famous essay "Power and Time," Mary Oliver writes that the greatest foe may not be the imperfect writing space or lack of inspiration. Our biggest foe as creative beings is our distracted mind. In pursuit of giving to others, we rob ourselves of our own creative energy. There are many ways to protect your energy. The idea here isn't to separate you from everyone else; we're not building a wall. Instead, imagine we are building a moat.

Moats are typically bodies of water surrounding a castle to provide protection and defense. The moat keeps some things out, but it also has bridges for others, even ideas, to enter the walls safely. You, and your writing practice, are the castle—now design a moat. Make it yours. Throw rose petals in it or anything else that brings you joy.

Write it!

Describe your moat.

On a New Narrative

Brenda Mitchell is an ordained pastor, state chapter coleader for Moms Demand Action in Illinois, senior fellow with Everytown Survivor Network, and member of Purpose Over Pain.

I'm equipped with the tools to guide me to my center. Pause allows me to take everything in my environment and stop it. I pause to recenter myself. I shut everything down, I close my eyes and I meditate and take a vacation with myself. I introduce myself to myself. I identify with my spiritual, my intellectual and ask to be brought back to a place where I can occupy my space. It still might be a little troubled, but I can still bring myself back to my center periodically in the day to continue my healing process in that moment.

Writing is a place of freedom for me. In order to free myself I first had to venture back into my past. It took me awhile to journey back to my past to look to that place where you no longer see yourself and revisit. Whatever you left there, salute it, understand it. That will actually free you.

I write, and I give myself away. Your life experiences are learned, and they're learned to be transformational. I've allowed my transformation and my hurt to lead others toward their healing process. People always talk about a new norm, but there are moments in life when you realize there will never be a new norm. I understand that.

With the death of my son, Kenneth, I realized that my life would never be the same and there would never be a new norm for me because normal was already out of my reach. Normal was the space that Kenneth occupied with us as a family. So, I will never have that level of happiness again because a piece of me is missing.

However, with meditation and with guidance through my healing and recovery process what I realized is that you can heal from trauma you just have to do the work. One of the biggest parts of this was not looking for a new norm.

What I realize is that I have created a new narrative for myself. In that new narrative, it's me. And in that new narrative I can find myself happy. A new narrative allows me a freedom that a new norm can't do for me. And Kenneth isn't left out of the process, Kenneth is the shaping of my new life that has allowed me to find happiness with and without him.

As I began this new narrative in my life, I began to put Kenneth in his proper position, never leaving him, but letting him occupy that space in my heart. That was a comfortable way for me to carry him and to continue on with the work. The work became helping someone else not have this experience became part of my healing. The more that I gave myself away the more healing that I experienced.

It took twelve years before I sought out this trauma healing. It took me four years to come through and get through it. It took me a long time to get through this because there were so many broken pieces of my life that I had just never touched, and I treated them like they had just never existed. I had to bring that all into focus along with my mourning process.

I choose to live so I'm not going to let death rule my life anymore. This is my mantra. It's scary sometimes, but I still choose to live.

Rewrite Your Story

I am not what happened to me, I am what I wish to become.
—Carl Jung, psychoanalyst

Writing a way forward can be a pathway out of trauma, a way to change history, a way to forge a future. When we've experienced a trauma, big or small, it means our brain doesn't comprehend time. Part of growing beyond your story means integrating it into a larger one of wellness. This applies to trauma stories and any other parts of our personal stories alike. This is also an effective way of moving any creative project along. This query inspires a fresh perspective of the moment.

Write it!

Instead of writing about what happened to you, write about what you choose to become. Write the version of you that you wish to see in five years (or even five minutes).

Joy Lives Within You, and It Is Your Right to Claim It

By moving from your outermost layers to the innermost layers, your truth is revealed; it will always rise to the top.

Sometimes when we're experiencing writer's block, it's because our stories are trapped in our bodies—locked in our joints, hiding in our organs, or lost in veins and passageways. One way to release them is to tap them out. Tapping your body can awaken the stories that need to speak and give you access to a source of infinite energy. I've learned different approaches to tapping and have used them in different contexts—there's not really a wrong way to do this. The idea is to pay attention and awaken the body by applying gentle taps with your palms or fingers along every surface.

This practice is invigorating, warming, and mood lifting. It can be done anytime, and it's especially suggested for winter months, when the body can be lethargic and withdrawn, or when you are experiencing other forms of lethargy, such as depression, stiffness, fear, or writer's block. Try it in silence. Try it with your favorite song.

Try it!

You may start standing or seated, depending on where you are with your body.

Begin standing with feet a little wider than hip-distance apart, with your knees slightly bent. If you're seated, bring your knees a little wider than your hips to create some space in the lower back and abdomen.

Lift both arms out in front of you, at shoulder height.

Bend your right elbow and bring your right palm (either stretched out flat or cupped) to your left arm and begin applying gentle taps to your outstretched left arm. Apply about the same amount of pressure you would if you were burping an infant.

Lightly tap up and down the arm, making sure to tap every centimeter of skin.

Tap with deliberate yet gentle action and find a consistent rhythm.

Switch arms and begin tapping the right arm.

In your own time, using both hands, move your tapping to the back of your shoulders and neck, across your upper chest and abdomen, and down your entire body.

Make gentle fists and bounce your hands off the sides of your hips and lower back. Don't forget your legs, ankles, and feet. Last, tap the top of your head, and with your awareness release any thoughts you no longer need.

At any point, pause and pay extra attention to any area of the body that needs it or enjoys it most.

When you're done, bring your arms along your sides and stand tall. You can bring your hands to your heart and belly, if you like.

Contemplate it!

Notice how you feel. What has changed? What has remained the same?

What's Your Headline?

You are the editor in chief of your life.

For my first job in publishing, I worked for an online news platform called Global Vision News Network. This was before the internet really took hold, and it was essentially an RSS feed that had affiliates with a few hundred international news stations. Each morning I had to handpick the five top stories in Western news outlets and then choose a number of stories from international sources related or not related to that headline. The idea was to show Western readers that there were other things going on in our world. What I got from this is that we shape our reality.

Each of us determines what is on our front page, what gets featured and what doesn't. Choose your headlines carefully. You will become what you share.

Write it!

If your life story was a news article, what would the headline be? Can you also name a few other headlines happening around the world that may or may not relate to yours?

Seek Boredom

Surprise! Boredom may be the touchstone to
all great creative breakthroughs.

Tibetan Buddhist meditation master Chogyam Trungpa separated
boredom into two kinds: cool and hot. Hot boredom can be understood like an itchy, hot potato kind of boredom. I liken this to a
roomful of teenagers at the end of a school day, moaning in frustra-
tion at how bored they are. They just *can't wait* to get out! Cool boredom is what happens when the thoughts begin to slow down.
Nothing is wildly interesting. Nothing is wildly boring. Things kind
of become as they are. And as they become as they are, we begin to
see more detail and experience the moment more fully, which allows
us to truly tap into a creative experience.

We don't necessarily want creativity to feel really exciting all the
time. When we're excited, we can't keep still. In order to write and
express our stories, we need to essentially cultivate this "boredom" so
we can access our senses.

Write it!

Write about a time you were bored. What were you doing, or, more
importantly, what weren't you doing? Maybe you're bored right now!
This is a great practice for waiting in line, in doctor's offices, or
whenever you're out of your normal routine. But you can also make
time to pursue boredom intentionally by putting it on your calendar
for this coming week.

What If?

Imagine the road not taken.

We all have experiences that we look back on and wonder what would have happened if we had made a different choice. Think of a time when you said no. What could have happened if you had said yes? This can be a rich creative playground.

Write it!

Write about a time you broke a pattern.

The Story of Your Breath

You can use your breath to drive your creative vision and path.

We all walk around with a reliable and powerful source that can bring us right into the present moment: our breath.

Right now, take a few deep breaths in and out, place your hands on your body, and listen for one minute.

What story does your breath have for you today? Is it long and smooth? Light and quick? Is your breath taking its time or in a rush?

Write it!

Personify your breath. Give your breath a name, personality, and occupation. What are its likes? Dislikes?

Ripple Effect

The language of empathy can spark widespread healing.

Tarana Burke created the Me Too movement in 2005 in Selma, Alabama, and began traveling around the country conducting workshops and panels to create a space for sexual violence survivors to connect with one another and make a statement to the world. In her memoir *Unbound: My Story of Liberation and the Birth of the Me Too Movement*, she writes, "What motivated me to continue were the little Black and Brown girls who trusted us with their secrets, their pain, their shame, their worries, their anger, their fears, and their hopes. It didn't take resources to introduce the possibility of healing into their lives. It didn't take wide-ranging support to stand them up. It took vision. It took intention. It took tenacity. It took courage. And it took empathy."[16]

Words can create a vibration that impacts our bodies. We see this in vibrational languages, like Sanskrit, where the meaning of the word is imbued in the vibrations of the sound. In some ways we can say this about all languages, including English, where the vibrations from language reverberate in our bodies. The words *me too* affect us on a cellular level. They can stimulate a relaxation response, which fosters resilience, connection, and a feeling of belonging.

In many ways *me too* can be thought of as the two most powerful words in the English language; these two words are another form of heart opening, an instant way to display empathy for one another.

Write it!

Reflect on a time that you gave or received the language of empathy. How did you feel inside? Write out the dialogue. How was empathy expressed? What is the language of empathy in your life?

What Story Do You Keep Telling Yourself?

Pause and bring to mind any stories that you are aware of that keep coming up again and again. Take a few moments to see them and welcome them. When you're ready, write them down if you wish. Choose any format or genre that you like; it could be a list, poem, letter, or news article.

Magical Objects

Everything has energy. Everything has a story.

One way to connect with inspiration is through objects. These include rocks, people, places, and things in our vicinity. Look around the room you are in. Notice the objects—the ones that are familiar to you and the ones that maybe you hadn't paid that much attention to before. Is one object capturing your imagination?

Write it!

Write the story of that object. Tell its origin story from the first-person perspective. If there are any people or animal friends nearby, you can feature them next. This is something you can try in both familiar and new places.

Host a Party for Your Thoughts

The only thing required is that you show up.

Ever wander out too far into a creative wilderness? Maybe you're stuck on a limb or at the end of a diving board or on a rooftop? This practice is another way to befriend your thoughts and reconnect with your creative flow.

The first time I taught this as a meditation, I emphasized too much how fun the party was going to be. This party doesn't need to be fun—it might be terrible, or it might be boring; guests you really wanted to hang out with might be no-shows. It's okay not to be able to plan for and predict everything. It's all part of the practice. It's all information.

This is a self-guided visualization practice; you might read through the instructions a few times first and then guide yourself, or record yourself and play it back. Take about five to ten minutes, depending on how long you want your party to be. Let your imagination lead the way.

Try it!

Find a comfortable seat and take a few rounds of breath.

Imagine your favorite place for a party. Imagine the location, the time of year. Are you outside or inside? Now begin to prepare for your party. Get dressed in your favorite party attire. Prepare any food or decorations. Do you need any help? Invite your favorite helpers. Now it's time for the party. Begin welcoming your guests. Your guests are your thoughts in your head. As they show up at the door of your mind (or maybe some just walk on in), welcome each one to the party. Observe how each guest appears. What do your thoughts look like? What are they wearing? How do they greet you? Give them names, bodies, characteristics. Focus on tending to your guests. What do they need to be comfortable? How are they doing? How are you doing? Remember, your helpers are here, so ask for their support as you need. Notice the buzz or flow or discomfort or conflict in the room of your mind. What is happening at your gathering? The party is now beginning to wind down. Help your guests gather their things. Say goodbye. Who leaves first? Who needs a gentle nudge to get on their way? It's time to clean up. Again, call on your helpers and observe the winding down.

Write it!

Describe what happened, the scene, and the guests.

Is There a Story You *Need* to Tell?

Stories are social change.

The silence of the written word is sometimes louder than a scream. You will know. You will feel it rumble. It can bubble up or evaporate, and it can erupt like a volcano. The march to create and share stories grows exponentially alongside every major social change.

Write about a time your voice felt like a roar.

On Creating Space from Your Story

Dan Cayer lives in the Hudson Valley and is writing a book about how to transform the experience of pain and illness into a path of openness and kindness.

My story is so personally meaningful to me, but what is important is to know that there are a lot of other stories out there. Don't think that your story is the only one. Also, don't think that adjacent stories are like yours. For example, I had an experience with disability, but that doesn't mean I know about other people's experiences with disability even though we may have some connection. Don't assume that just because you are writing about trauma that you understand others.

Writing about the experience made it about a thing that happened to me, and I was involved in, but it wasn't the essential outcome, I didn't choose it. I think a lot of people who have chronic pain and things like that, think there can be kind of a sense of failure, especially if your condition is not extremely clear cut. Oh, for me, writing about it, it was like, "Oh, so here's this twenty-five-year-old kid, and he's working at this company and this thing happened," and I could think, "Oh, that was really hard." In some ways it was like the role of a therapist.

The first draft was only part of the distancing. It was also really helpful to edit that stuff out. The editing was actually really healthy. It's about care for the reader, and it is also really good to realize, "Oh, I don't need to say that. I don't need to go into this long, drawn-out worker's compensation experience that was hellish. I don't need to bring people through it." And that helped me let go of it. I don't need to carry this material with me forever. Unless it's helping or working for me. I don't need to carry it.

As an Alexander Technique teacher, one thing I found is people often think the worst part of their chronic pain is their pain, and it can be, but when you have a more reflective practice, whether it's meditation or writing, it's often these things that the pain results in, like shame. Like in my case, shame over not being able to work, or to be able to help my wife, or the pain results in this tremendous sense of no control over your life. You wake up and you think, I have no idea what I'm going to be able to do today or what it's going to be like." Or you feel more distant from other people, because they don't understand how difficult it is to just go to the grocery store and shop. Writing can help you understand what's going on at a deeper level beyond your back pain or your neck pain. It will help you understand the dynamics underneath that are probably being revealed in this. Like a sense of helplessness, which is horrible. Or a sense of I'm inferior to other people because of . . . These are the kinds of things that are always there in one way or another in chronic pain. Culturally we only care about what you are doing to fix it.

My go-to [prompt] forever has been to keep the hand moving and follow what's interesting. Sometimes a good prompt is "What's the hardest part about this?"

Write it!

Describe the hardest part. Welcome any stress or pain. Perhaps you're experiencing pain right now, either acute or chronic. Or perhaps you have a memory of a pain in the body. Tell the story of either what happened or what the pain has to say. What's the hardest part? What does it have to say?

What Do You *Need* to Tell Your Story?

Treat your story like a start-up.

So many creative souls relegate their work to the seams and cracks of their lives—the wee hours of the morning, the corner of a messy table. We imagine ourselves to be like cacti, only needing sporadic droplets of nourishment to survive. We all know these are not the best conditions for the kind of healing writing we are talking about.

What kind of support do you need to make this creative expression possible? What if you began this process with these conditions in place so you can thrive?

Write it!

Make your list of what you need—try to be specific:

Time?

Space?

Money?

Food?

Coaching?

Emotional support?

Therapy?

Research?

Supplies?

A babysitter?

Keep going . . .

Invite Your Reader to the Page

Writing doesn't have to be lonely and isolating.

It may be helpful to invite the spirit of your future readers when you sit down to write. They can guide your voice and inspire content. They can keep you company. This doesn't mean you're sharing anything at this point. This is purely an energetic invitation.

Name up to three people you *actually* know whom you'd want to have in your energetic space right now. These entities could be your pet, your friend, your boss, or a younger version of you. It can be nice to keep a photo of them nearby or something of meaning that reminds you of them.

Write it!

Describe these people, like you're writing a profile on them. Where do they live? How old are they? What are their likes and dislikes? What is their favorite color, food? Who are they? Do a thorough character study of them, as if you were describing them to a reporter.

Surround Yourself
with Beautiful Language

Beauty is an action, it is nourishment, it is fuel.

The best way to create beautiful language is to experience beautiful language. You don't need to do anything with it; just be with it. Like the sun, it will cloak you with a warmth that will give you a creative glow, boost your mood and energy, and offer unexpected inspiration.

What this means is tending to and feeding your inner writer with inspiring books, poetry, podcasts, and other literary delights.

Take a moment and reflect on your reading practice. What does it look like? How often do you read? What does it feel like when you read?

Try it!

Read a poem first thing in the morning for the next two weeks, before looking at your phone. Journal about how it affects your day. If poetry isn't your thing, choose a song or an excerpt from another piece of writing.

Describe the Light

Wherever you are right now, the way the light is currently falling will never happen in exactly the same way again.

One thing we can rely on is that the light will change. For that reason, describing the light is always a great way to get present and begin a practice.

Write it!

Look around and observe where the light is coming from and where it is falling. Describe the light around you now—whether it's natural light, candlelight, a lamp, or even the halo from technology. Write about what it looks like, feels like, how it's affecting the surroundings. What is it helping you see? Does this light remind you of anything?

Mindful Eavesdropping

Paying attention establishes safety in your environment and is a powerful key to sourcing creative material.

When I was about twelve years old and reaching a peak of adolescent angst—the "door slamming, clove cigarettes, dying my hair, piercing body parts" stage—my aunt Abby took me on a vacation to Disney World. Over a spaghetti dinner, she turned to me and said, "Okay, Lisa, I'm about to teach you a very important life lesson. I'm going to teach you how to eavesdrop."

I was spellbound. She continued in great detail and care, instructing me in the art of eavesdropping.

"The most important part," she said, "is to not make it too obvious that you're eavesdropping. Try to fit in and relax into your environment . . . You just have to wait and pick up bits of conversation here and there. It can help to look occupied and like you are enjoying yourself so people don't know you are listening." She concluded by saying, "Once you learn how to do this, you'll never be bored."

We spent the rest of that meal, and every other meal for the remainder of the vacation, in silence, looking like we were enjoying each other's company and listening. Every now and then, I would nod at her and report my findings. "That man just told his wife that his sister is having an affair" or "That kid is getting in so much trouble!" or "That man is going to propose." My aunt would be thrilled! "Good job, Lisa." She'd smile so hard tears formed in her eyes. "You have a knack for this! I taught you well."

I'm relieved because I have something to talk about and a way to connect with the environment around me. I walked away from this trip with a new superpower, the ability to cultivate curiosity in others wherever I am. Knowing who's around me helps me find safety in my space and sparks inspiration. Every voice is new material. In retrospect it was my first mindfulness listening meditation.

Try it!

Go outside and find a public space you can hang out in for a bit—a coffee shop, park bench, train station; you choose. Listen and take note of great dialogue. Begin a new story with a line you hear. Find your next story.

You can use this same technique with books, poetry collections, newspapers, podcasts. Open up your favorite novel, poetry collection, or newspaper—anything you have around that's written. Choose a line that speaks to you. Begin a new piece with that line.

Between Places

Judith Hannan teaches writing about personal experience to homeless mothers and at-risk adolescents as well as to medical professionals and students; she is a writing mentor with the Visible Ink program, which serves patients at the Memorial Sloan-Kettering Cancer Center. She is the author of *The Write Prescription* and *Motherhood Exaggerated*.

I thought of the image of a bridge when I was trying to figure out where I was in my own life, which was full of transitions at the time. By using metaphor, I was able to get a clearer picture of what was before and behind me, what was blocking me and what was urging me on, in what ways I was being supported and how I was being undermined. The bridge is never the same. This can be a prompt to return to often.

Close your eyes and imagine a bridge.

Write it!

Describe the bridge.

Celebrate Your Resilience

The only way to truly see where you are going
is to recall where you've been.

Recall a challenge you had six months ago that you thought you
would never overcome.

Write it!

Write about how you overcame it.

Music Heals and Reveals

A song can inspire a full-body response and coax our nervous system back in time to a particular time and place.

Some writers I've worked with insist on absolute silence, others prefer the hum of a coffee shop, and a few like to have music playing in the background. Whatever your preferred environment, it's indisputable that music offers a unique opportunity to tap into inspiration and deep healing. Listening to a familiar song can be a powerful way to time travel, lift your mood, and shift your perspective and creative experience.

Many of us know on a gut level that listening to music can make us feel better, even make us want to move. Music also has powerful, deep, and lasting healing properties that can have a measurable impact on your health and well-being. Recent studies from the Johns Hopkins Medicine Center for Music and Medicine show listening to music regularly can reduce anxiety and depression; it can be good for your heart, reduce pain, and even have a positive effect on patients who have experienced strokes and dementia.

Take a moment to acknowledge how good it is for you to listen to music. Recalling the benefits of a practice before diving in can amplify its healing capacity.

Try it!

This exercise will require a music source, so go grab your phone, computer, stereo, or instrument. This can be a great prompt to try when you are digging deeper into a scene and searching for more description.

Think of your favorite song from a pivotal moment in your life—for example, the year you were thirteen, the first time you tried something, or perhaps a time you needed comfort. Any memorable moment will work.

Now, play that song (literally).

As you're listening, close your eyes and breathe with the sound. Notice the images, shapes, or smells that pop up. It doesn't have to be anything complex or hidden, and it may affect you in ways that you're not immediately aware of.

Modification

Focus on the vibrations you feel within or outside, either when music is playing or not.

Write it!

Free write about the associations, memories, and sensations that come up. Reflect on what has changed and what has remained the same since you listened to the song.

Write About Grapefruit

Sometimes the best way into a creative practice is to describe ordinary objects and experiences, such as describing a grapefruit or the food you ate for breakfast. Letting go of the bigger questions and goals and feelings helps you focus on what's right in front of you and what you can hold.

Write it!!

Write about a grapefruit (or if you prefer, write about your breakfast experience today).

Childhood Kitchen

Think back to a meaningful kitchen from your childhood. It could be from your own household, someone else's, or another place where cooking happened.

Write it!

Describe the kitchen.

Shake Break

Take a moment for movement.

Stretch your fingers out in front of you. Observe their magnificence.
Now, shake, shake, shake! Fan your face with your delicious fingers and move your hands every which way.
When you're done, thank your hands.

Modification

Imagine a wind shaking loose any stories that are stuck to you.

Memories

Notice the stories you carry and how they define who you are.

Our sense of self is a construct made up of narratives we tell ourselves and others. The stories you carry are made up of your own experiences, memories, instincts, and beliefs. They may also be made up of stories other people told you or ones you were born with. The prompts below are designed to be sparks to help you get more personal with the stories you are holding by mining your own memory. You can play around with changing how you tell the story to change your sense of who you are.

Read through the list, choose the one that resonates most now, and write.

Describe your first frenemy.

Describe an animal that had meaning for you.

Describe your first school.

Describe a time that you lied.

Describe your sixteenth birthday.

Describe your first drink.

Describe your first kiss.

Describe a grandparent.

Describe your first big failure.

Describe your first big success.

Describe an embarrassing story.

Name four more that I left out.

Write Around the Wound

Learning to write from the eye of the storm.

Sometimes we have a burning urge to write in the middle of a traumatic, life-changing moment. This could look like a major emotional turmoil or chronic illness; it could also be an assault or violation or major milestone, like getting sober, leaving a marriage, moving, or any other out-of-the-ordinary experiences. We also get this urge when really joyful and exciting things happen. While writing can be a helpful tool for self-care, soothing, and clarifying, it's hard, maybe impossible, to write *well* in the middle of a frenzy.

When you're right in the middle of the chaos of a challenging time, writing directly about your challenge isn't always healthy or fruitful. It's easy to get too close and lost in the shadows of the story as it's playing out—poking the fresh wound rather than giving it space to heal. I've seen time and time again, both in my own experience and working with others, how writing about a trauma as it is happening can deepen the intensity of feeling rather than provide grounding and perspective. It takes time to process and sift through complicated emotional experiences. I've learned that writing around the wound or adjacent to it brings about more comfort, healing, and better, more evocative writing.

Here are a few ways to work with a challenge while it is happening:

Make It Fiction

If you know you are writing about difficult emotions or a traumatic incident, try *not* writing about it directly. Free your grip on the details of the incident by changing a key element of the story (when it happened, the point of view, or where it happened). Be gentle. You also may learn more about the true impact of the event on your spirit and find some better language for expressing what happened and how you feel about it. Writing as fiction will help you create more empathy for yourself.

You don't need to add magic or fairies or anything outlandish to make it fiction; just change one feature, such as

- age
- occupation
- gender
- race
- location
- nationality

Change something significant about the story—like the point of view or time period—or change the incident entirely.

Time Is a Tool

Instead of writing in the present tense, choose a time many months (or even years) before the incident and write about a benign moment. If time has passed since the incident, you can shoot ahead in time and write about many seasons later. You will still explore the themes and emotions you want to because this is you writing, but the tool of time will allow you to write more richly, and you will have more access to details and descriptions.

Just the Facts

What's important during these times, these times that you know you'll want to write about at some point, is to help yourself remember and record. For a week, keep a fact-based journal. What this means is that you'll jot down everything you take in with your senses, just the facts, no emotions—what you actually see, hear, smell, taste, or feel. Avoid using reflective language or analysis or feeling. Simply make a list of what happened using the same tone, thoroughness, and clarity that you might offer a court of law.

Nourish

Take a few breaths here.

Let's take a self-care break. Do you need some water? A snack? Do you need to refresh yourself? Stretch?

Describe a Body Part

Invite your body to the page.

Your body may appreciate a little VIP treatment and attention; give it a personalized invitation. Invite your body to the page by writing about it.

Try it!

Choose a body part that is uncomfortable right now, and describe it.

Choose a body part that is pain-free right now, and describe it.

Choose a body part you feel neutral about or a part you've been ignoring, and describe it.

Shopping List

Offer your creative life the same time and effort as your body and home.

Pause for a moment and write down your weekly grocery list. That's right. Go ahead and think about what food you need for the day or the week ahead.

When was the last time you put that much thought into planning your creative life?

So many of us spend years nursing a dream about pursuing a creative life. But when it's actually within our reach, we shrink. We go shopping, clean the house, walk the dog, take a drink, eat something, call someone, scroll on our phones—anything but write.

Today, stay.

Write it!

Write down your goals for your creative life this week.

Let Your Senses Speak

What have you observed since waking up this morning?

Make a list of at least seven things you have observed since waking up this morning. You can swap around the senses here too; there are no rules for how you experience the senses. Describe what you

- saw
- heard
- smelled
- touched
- tasted

Hero's Journey

Return to your hero's journey.

Try writing from a place of pride and accomplishment. All hero's journeys, from *The Odyssey* to *The Wizard of Oz* to *Their Eyes Were Watching God*, have the same main components. A main character in distress goes out into the world seeking meaning; after conquering a challenge, they return transformed, and they *almost always* return to someone in order to share their message (and love). What journey are you on? What message do you have for the world? Who do you want to return to?

Write it!

Write a story with you as the hero.

Begin Again

Every time we face a new page, we have the chance to reorient our thoughts.

We all have days that just don't go as planned. Conversations go awry. The train doesn't come on time. We often don't have any control over this. We might have done everything right, eaten the right thing, exercised, been of service, and yet . . . and yet still your favorite class was canceled, or you ran out of milk, or you feel uninspired and have nothing to write.

Or you said exactly the wrong thing.

You have a choice in a moment like this. You can ruminate and fester, or you can begin again.

Starting again offers the promise of a new perspective, a new experience. This can begin with the breath. Each inhale is a new start. Writing also allows us to begin again.

Write it!

Tell a story and then begin again. Tell it a different way. Repeat until you have three versions of the same story, each with a new beginning, middle, and end.

Coax Your Voice

Get your story to come to you.

Ever go to a party and get cornered by someone who just can't stop talking?

They talk about all kinds of things—they talk about themselves, their accomplishments, their thoughts, and their path. They may also pepper you with questions about your background, your job, your pet, your personal life. This, of course, is another way of them talking about themselves because they are controlling the direction and rhythm of the conversation.

Meanwhile, your back is pinned against the wall, your breath is shallow, and you offer short phrases and single-word answers and a tense nod to try to push them back. Instead of listening, you're strategizing how the hell you are going to get out of there. You have no new ideas, nothing to add, no nuance to offer. You might wonder where your personality is.

This is how your story feels when you are overcrowding and suffocating it. It has no place to go. You need to carve out a listening space within you for your story to fill.

Step away from whatever you are writing and let a story—the one you have been trying to write or a different one—come to you.

Write it!

Personify your story. How would it behave at a party? Give it a name, an identity, likes, dislikes. Give your story enough space to surprise you.

You Are the Inspiration You Seek

What you seek is seeking you.

—Rumi

So much of being a writer is harnessing inspiration. We travel the world, take courses, buy books, go on intensive self-improvement explorations ad infinitum. We go to great lengths to get lost in the wilderness, only to find that everything we are seeking is within.

Write it!

Make a list of qualities you possess that inspire you. This could include experiences you've gathered, kindness you've given, or art you've made. Start with something small, like making your bed, and go from there.

Hug

Try it!

Stretch your arms out into a T shape and then wrap them around yourself. Rock a little side to side. Hold tight, but not too tight. Take five breaths.

This practice ensures that you get at least one great hug today.

PART FOUR

Inspire

TIGHTROPE WALKER

Barely four feet tall, I float thirty feet above the ground. I spend my days confidently placing one foot in front of another on a razor-thin wire.

I hold my center and take a step out, trusting the next step will come. My strong feet grip the rope. The rope bounces, and inside a part of me squeals. My body exhales as I bend my knees slightly, and my hips sway a little, almost like a dance. I take another step and steady myself. I do this again and again, never taking my eyes off the rope in front of me. *Keep going.* Eventually I get to the other side and realize I am smiling. From below I hear clapping and a counselor shouts, "You're a natural!" I am on top of the world—literally—feeling myself but not by myself.

In fourth grade, we move from a progressive neighborhood in Manhattan to a small village flanked by three churches and a football field known for its fine school system and strong antisemitic past. My first week of school during dodgeball, I heckle the others; however, instead of a choir of rowdy schoolmates joining me, a teacher whisks toward me and whispers in my ear, "I don't know where you're from, but here girls don't talk that way."

A week later, when I'm leaving school, I feel a few hot stings against my back. At first, I think I have been stung by a bee, but then I hear a few boys chanting, "Jew! Jew! Pick it up! Jew! Jew! Pick it up!" They are singing and throwing pennies at me.

I think, *But I'm not even Jewish. I'm half Welsh!* An instinct to be polite takes over. I bend down and pick up the coins one by one and walk over to the leader and hand them to him. "Are these yours?" I don't tell anyone what had happened to me, and a new hard feeling plants itself in my gut.

I feel out of place, and a voice inside tells me to run with that; I quickly *make sure* I don't fit in. I fashion myself as different in every way I can. I wear summer clothes in winter, winter clothes in summer; I give myself a startling haircut, cutting my bangs a millimeter long in an ahead-of-its-time style.

During home ec, a fifties-era class designed to teach us how to become homemakers, instead of following directions and sewing a skirt, I design a huge pair of sweatpants and write "give peace a chance" in bubble paint down the legs. In the following weeks, I become a one-woman protest of the Iraq War up and down the hallways.

The following summer, my parents send me to circus camp. Allegedly, they don't really know it's circus camp—it's a performance art camp, which happens to have fire eating and juggling options for activities. My dad is at the wheel for the bucolic two-hour drive; he tries to talk to me while I listen to my Walkman, head down. "If you only knew how lucky you are," my mother says on my departure, which I answer with a silent single word: *shutupihateyou.*

I arrive at camp braced to defend and judge before others have the chance to judge me. My father walks quickly ahead of me, as if he knows the way, carrying my large duffle bag packed full of books. It's weird to see a New Yorker in the wild. He looks somehow shorter, browner, and skinnier than I know him to be. His fast, purposeful movements are out of sync with the pace of trees.

I trail behind when a strawberry-blonde teenager bounces up to us. "Lisa? I'm Jamie! I'm your bunk leader!" The cheeriness of her voice startles me like a bright flashlight. I take note of her thick, rainbow-colored braided anklet; faded baby-blue short-shorts; and worn-in penny loafers—a stark contrast to my checkered turquoise-and-black knee-length jams and black high-top sneakers. I bite my nails. She takes us on a tour starting with a mess of small bunks. It is like a tiny city. Around the bend is a lake; a few preppy kids giddily play some sort of game in the water. I have never seen it before—they are yelling out, "Marco!" and "Polo!" and Jamie says, "They're playing Marco Polo."

"That looks fun, Lisa!" my dad says, too loudly, like I am six years old. I roll my eyes, look down, and nod, trying my best to disappear. Jamie points out various other attractions, like the theater and cafeteria. I hear my mom's voice—"I would have killed to have an opportunity like this when I was your age." After the art studios, Jamie pauses and raises her arms to the right in delight. Looming over the entire camp is a huge circus tent. Like a marionette, I shift my gaze toward my dad; his face opens into a wide smile. "Dad, did you know about this?" He shrugs.

I am incredulous. How had I not heard of this part?! I am both scared and intrigued. Maybe the summer won't be as bad as I thought. I spend the first week excusing myself at every opportunity from activities that intimidate me. Most campers have set their sights on prestigious plays and rigorous studio-art experiences, which I'm not qualified for or interested in. I secretly feel drawn to the circus. I know I am most comfortable doing the most uncomfortable thing. It feels like a place I can be me.

The morning of tryouts, I feel led as I tiptoe over to the circus tent. A little voice says, *Go.* Inside, a world of chaos unfolds. I pace from booth to booth, my body tight with worry and anguish. In one corner are the clowns. They already look like they belong to each other—like a family unit caked in makeup and ecstatic, painted-on laughter. *Was I the kind of person who could be a clown—loud, funny, and outrageous?*

I clench my sweaty hands into fists waiting in line to audition. When I get closer to the front of the line, I hear the head clown say, "Make a joke! Then laugh!" to the camper in front of me. *Whoa, no way. I can't laugh on command.* An inner voice tells me, *Slowly back away, nice and easy.* I feel my hair growing frizzier by the minute with the summer heat.

As I maze around the crowded tent to survey the remaining options, I look up and spot the trapeze. I think, *That! That's hard. I can do that.* Watching Stacy—a popular girl with long silky brown hair—high above the ground swinging, being caught, and nearly missing makes my heart flip with excitement. *Yes, yes, yes.* I skip to the audition line.

But it is too late. They are full.

Nearly defeated, I notice out of the corner of my eye a vibrant kerfuffle going on just outside the tent. Curious, I walk over to the small group of misfit campers. *Are these my people?* Their eyes are glued to an enthusiastic adult pointing with a long rod. I, too, follow the rod with my eyes and find myself looking up, up, up toward a thin line suspended in midair: the tightrope.

"You!" he yells, pointing at me.

Startled, I crane my neck and see two poles with a thin wire strung between them. The sun is in my eyes, making them tear.

"You!" He points at me again. "You're small. You'll be perfect!"

I notice the other kids smiling. And just like that, I belong.

———

The tightrope is thirty feet above ground and about twenty feet long. Every day for the rest of the summer, a harness is attached to my waist, and I am hoisted up to the ledge where the tightrope is attached. As I ascend, I dissolve into the rush and relief of being alone in the quiet vastness. Once I steady myself on the stand, I look out across the camp, which has grown smaller, farther away, and friendlier. My heart pounds in my chest with anxiety and excitement and then slows to an easy *lub-dub* voice. Even the sky, the clouds, the sun feel like friends, coconspirators on this new adventure.

A gentle voice from within says, *Walk.* So I do.

I have a full schedule the rest of the summer. I spend the mornings dodging camp activities and each afternoon quietly putting one foot in front of the other midair. I escape into the discipline. When I am on the rope, I ignore how it cuts into my foot, and all of my shame, insecurities, fears, and anger disappear. I am laser focused, following a steady inner voice: *Hold your head high, lengthen your spine, breathe deeply, and look straight ahead.* I never quite know when the rope will bounce or sway, whether a sharp gust of wind will knock me over.

About a week later, the instructor removes the safety ropes and gives me a six-foot-long pole to hold as I walk. It is quite heavy, and it seems crazy that adding weight will make life easier—but it does; it helps me balance. I learn how to adjust my pace, walking faster and slower and with a little bit of rhythm, like a song from within. I learn I am stronger than I think I am when I move *with* the wire. I learn how to walk looking straight ahead at the horizon rather than down at the wire and how to relax my feet and narrow my peripheral vision, which had the potential to send me tumbling into the abyss.

For the circus finale, I wear a simple black outfit, tank top and shorts, with my hair pulled into a high ponytail, no frills, no bows. I arrive early, barefoot and alert, to observe the expected crowd. There are about thirty people assembled. My family decides to skip the show. I swallow and tell myself, *I'm not doing this for them; my audience is within.*

For one last time, I am hoisted up. When I get to the ledge, I notice the staff has removed the safety net beneath me for the performance. Now my only protection is the rope attached to my small waist. Someone must have told me this before, but I have forgotten. A flame of fear whips up my spine. We have practiced this final trick a few times in the previous weeks. I hear a voice say, "You got this."

I walk out to the center of the wire. I kneel, curl up like a little human bowling ball, and hold very still. Next, the counselor—and all 130 pounds of his teenage frame—walks toward me from the other end of the rope. I must stay very still and very low so the rope doesn't shake. While he walks, I count my breath and hope (well, maybe I pray too) he won't fall.

When he reaches me in the center, I feel him push off the rope and arc over me. First, I brace myself, and then I remember to relax, to move with the rope—we both need it to sway with our weight, if we don't want to fall. When he lands like a cat on the other side, the rope bounces, and he bounces, and I am sure we will fall, even though we never fell in all the times we practiced.

At the moment my fear peaks, the rope shakes beneath us, and as I take a breath, I find my center and hold it until the rope eventually stops shaking. As the rope settles, my confidence remains.

Find Inspiration

Up until this point, you have been cultivating and nourishing an inward journey. In the following pages, we'll explore *how* to make that leap from internal to external. Every creator, every writer, needs to find a sense of belonging in the world that's not dependent on another human being in order to release their work. That is where creative courage comes from. The next step in this journey is connecting with an energy that will propel, guide, and support you through the process of unveiling the story you are now meant to share.

How Do You Find Inspiration?

There are as many ways to find inspiration as there are humans on this planet. The path is personal, roomy, and vast. For some this might be a higher power, or higher self; it can be a spiritual connection; it can be beauty; it can also be called God; it can be your reader or one of your characters; it can be your ancestors or nature or music; it can be any number of things. I have a close friend who refers to their source as Wonder Woman. Lean in to what works to expand your creative vision.

For some, the writing practice itself, the repetition, the discipline, the ritual, creates a spiritual experience. In the yoga tradition, and many other spiritual traditions, there's an understanding that consistent practice, over a long period of time and in earnest effort, will yield inspiration. Since we have just practiced writing in the last chapter, perhaps you're already feeling some of this.

We all have a limitless supply of inspiration within, but we don't always have access to it. There are many ways to invite in, seek out, and connect with an inspiration source. Inspiration will come, eventually, when you seek it. It may even come in the form of writer's block, which forces us to pause and slow down. Everything and anything can be a spark when you are available to it.

Why We Need Inspiration

We all get stuck, we all encounter obstacles, and we all feel alone. Obstacles and roadblocks can come in many forms, such as societal oppression, illness, or impostor syndrome, and they can also come in the form of writer's block, dullness, and boredom. Inspiration is what can lift us up and return us to our path. It is a reliable place to return to and reconnect with our purpose, to refuel.

What are some ways that you find meaning and direction? Do you connect in nature, movement, animals, water, wind? Do you connect with a person, a guide, or an ancestor? Your own breath can be a form of spiritual connection; the rhythm of your breath can be your guide. The word *inspire* comes from the Latin word *inspirare*, which means to blow into or breathe on. Another word that means breath is *spirit*. Which means, in a sense, you can breathe in spirit or that you need to (pause and) breathe to find inspiration. We have done some breathing already on this path.

Whatever you choose, inspiration needs to be something you can really feel and connect with. You can change as you go; just begin with something that feels right. What matters most is that it's something that works for you, something that's just yours and that you can rely on any time of day—no matter what is going on around you.

This force may come from someplace else, but the voice you are seeking is your own. This connection will always lead you back to your authentic voice.

Your Inner GPS

If our inner GPS leads us around, then our
stories are our maps.

We each have our own compass, or inner GPS system, which is
designed for each one of us alone. It's a perfect fit for your body, and
when you're feeling safe and connected, it's easy to follow that compass and know where you're supposed to go, who you're supposed to
be, and what you're supposed to say, create, do, and write. When our
bodies are frozen, tense, or afraid, we can lose this connection,
meander along the way, and get off course.

However, even a GPS system or compass doesn't operate on its
own. It orients around a destination and corrects as it goes. It can
follow bread crumbs, signposts, and stars along the way.

Write it!

Describe your compass. Where is it situated? Where does your compass needle point?

On Inspiration

Stephen Cope is a best-selling author and scholar who specializes in the relationship between the Eastern contemplative traditions and Western depth psychology. Among his seminal works in this area are *Yoga and the Quest for the True Self*, *The Wisdom of Yoga*, and *The Great Work of Your Life*.

I call my books dharma assignments. I don't launch forward on a big project until I have a clear assignment from the universe. It becomes clear over a period of time what is being called for. I don't always understand why that's being called for now. It certainly doesn't come from me. And that's my work until it's finished.

I follow what I call the brail method which is listening to my guidance one step at a time. My motto is suit up and show up, I have an agreement with myself that I show up every morning. I show up at my computer and if I don't want to write, I don't have to, because I need to be in the right frame of mind. I almost never don't want to write.

My next motto is move the marbles forward just a little bit every day. Just move it forward a little bit. Let go of big plans and schemes. Let go of I'm going to get a Pulitzer with this project. Just thinking of the small as large. I listen to my inspiration; I listen to my guides, and I dive into the writing. This is not a linear process at all. You don't know why you need to go through writing this chapter to get to this chapter. And then that previous chapter gets thrown on the floor. It happens all the time. And it requires a massive amount of trust. It requires quiet, listening, trusting the voices you hear. And that's not only the voices I get in my own head, but I do a tremendous amount of sharing of my material with people I trust. If you have one person like that, it's golden, especially if that person is a good reader.

The idea is what arises in you (if you're really a writer) are occasional hints and hunches and little visions and little desires inside about what you would like to write about, what you need to write about. They come at first in these hunches and intuitions, and then very often they go away, and they come back, and they go away, and they come back and then something begins to sound like a melody. It sounds like something real that you want to reach for.

Gratitude Seeker

It's possible to reprogram your default setting.

Once a traumatic memory gets stored, our librarian brain archives it by theme (e.g., feelings of loneliness, feelings of isolation, misunderstanding, or being trapped). And over time, whenever we have another experience that is similar, we feel all those past emotions again, amplified. We learn to turn to those stories as our defaults. As we tell and retell these stories to ourselves, we become convinced this is our worldview, just the way we are. As we recover, we can adjust our worldview without erasing or denying any painful memories by filling our brain with another powerful narrative structure, like gratitude. We can tell a new story, and retell it, and retell it, until it becomes the new default story and offers a radical shift in perspective.

A few years ago, when I was feeling particularly stuck and isolated (two of my go-to old stories), a friend invited me to join a gratitude list with a few people. She told me to try to contribute ten things I was grateful for every day. The whole idea made me uncomfortable, but I decided to give it a go. The first time I sat down to write my list, I couldn't think of a single thing. The lists I was accustomed to either itemized tasks that needed to be completed or were things I disliked and wanted to improve about myself—who I was, where I lived, what I did, how I felt, what I lacked . . .

I felt lost, so I went on a walk to look for something to be grateful for. As I walked, I started noticing things—the sound of a child laughing, the sun dancing on the river, the many shades of green on a tree. These observations stirred something in me. Those three things were the first three items on my first list. I oriented the rest of my day looking for more experiences I could be grateful for. Then I did it again the next day, the day after that, and so on. Over time, I started to think of myself as a gratitude seeker. The more I did it, the easier it became to find things to be grateful for.

A practice of gratitude is like a salute to the presence of some kind of benevolent force or greater energy.

I'll offer a few ways to walk into gratitude, and you'll find your own way.

But first, I'm grateful for you.

Try it!

Peruse these suggestions for gratitude inspiration and write a list that feels aligned with your style.

Who Helped?

Who helped get you here? This could be a spirit guide, animal guide, or an ancestor. It could even be someone right now, today, who is helping you make space to try this practice—maybe they are taking care of your cat, or child, or dog, or maybe they gave you this book as a gift. Offer them thanks.

Write it!

Write them a thank-you letter. Send it.

If they are no longer with us, you can send it to their loved ones or ceremonially address it and bury or burn it.

What Are You Grateful for in Your Body? In Your Mind? Spirit?

Write it!

Make a list.

From the Future

Bring to mind anything you are worried about or anything you are *pining* for!

Write a gratitude from some far future place, from a perspective when those things have been resolved or acquired. How do you imagine they got resolved? What do you imagine you have acquired, accomplished, or received?

Further Suggestions

Notice your physical surroundings; what are you grateful for?
Who are you grateful for?
Are there any people in your life, currently or in the past, who you're grateful for?
Are there any foods or activities you're enjoying? You can be grateful for those.
What successes are you grateful for?
What failures are you grateful for?
Any challenges? Opportunities to grow?
What have you forgotten to be grateful for?
Keep going . . .

Fill Up Your Cup

You can't give what you do not possess.

Medical studies far and wide—ranging from Dr. Rita Charon's seminal program in Narrative Medicine at Columbia University to similar subsequent programs at Yale University, Mass General, University of Wisconsin, and others—have shown that a creative writing practice can offer meaningful improvement in doctors' well-being and ability to cope with their work and offer quality care. These writing programs can help to support doctors' emotional burdens. In many of these classes, students read a wide range of literary texts and are given writing assignments relating to their medical practice and general creative practice. The programs provide meaningful emotional support for their work in and out of the field of medicine. There are similar writing programs offered to patients at places like Sloane Kettering, Cedars Sinai, and others. Through this work, a new literary art has been born, and over the years journals such as *Bellevue Literary Review*, *Intima: A Journal of Narrative Medicine*, and *Visible* have emerged to publish illness stories by doctor and patient alike.

Whether you are a professional caregiver, medical practitioner, healing-arts professional, teacher, friend, assistant, manager, neighbor, mother, father, sister, daughter, or son, chances are there is someone or something under your care on a regular basis. A writing practice can be a way to replenish your energies so you have more to give.

Write it!

Write about a time writing has helped you process a difficult experience.

Who Is Your Authentic Voice?

Before you step out into the world to share your story, you first need to truly feel heard and held.

Who do you turn to when no one else is around? Who cheers you on when you're afraid you might fall? Can you summon this voice? It can be someone imagined, no longer with us, or out of reach. It doesn't need to be a real person. Your authentic voice lives within you. This voice is always leading you where you need to go. You are never alone.

Write it!

Describe your authentic voice. What does it sound like? Look like? Is it in human form? If so, does it have a favorite outfit or age? What is its pronoun? Race? Nationality? Be specific. Make it personal.

Design a Safe Place

Give your mind a place to rest and return to.

What does *feeling safe and relaxed* mean to you? For so many of us, it doesn't even feel safe to feel safe. Whatever kind of trauma you are living with, it's natural and wise to walk around with a certain tension and suspicion, like you're walking on eggshells.

Various therapeutic modalities work with the concept of creating a soothing safe place with your imagination before diving into deeper layers of psychological work, especially relating to challenging emotional work and trauma. This method can be really useful when you're writing about difficult topics, including trauma. It can give you a place to rest and reset, and it can also help you create a neutral space to invite a future reader or listener into.

Try it!

Close your eyes and imagine your favorite place. This can be real or imagined. Pick someplace where you feel safe, secure, and enjoy being. It can be outside or inside. Other people and animals can be there, or you can be on your own. Spend a few minutes imagining this place and see yourself in it.

Write it!

What do you see? What does it feel like to be there?

Two-Way Listening

Using your imagination and spiritual
connection, actively invite your inner guide to
join you.

You don't need a living, breathing mortal in front of you to find connection. Another way to invite your creative muse in is through a
two-way writing practice. The idea is to invite spirit to commune
with you, like a cowriter or copilot. There are many layers of sharing
that happen before you share with another person, let alone a
stranger. This can be one.

Begin by finding a quiet place and connecting to your breath.
Meditate for a few minutes and listen.

Write it!

You can practice this on the page by asking a question and then
waiting for an answer. Some people like to practice this by using
their nondominant hand for the answers. Try it any way you like.

1. Write a line or a question.
2. Wait for a response or imagine a response.
3. Continue in this back-and-forth way for ten minutes.

On Some Guiding Principles

Brette Popper is a yoga teacher and writer.

There is a desire in the culture I've been exposed to that you do something once and all of a sudden, you're supposed to be an expert at it. Even in the yoga world, you can see people going out and getting a two-hundred-hour certificate and they're supposed to go out and teach. This desire to be an expert immediately or have a coat of wisdom out of whatever you're doing is not instant or immediate by any circumstances. It takes a lot of time. It takes a long, long time. Whether it's doing a physical practice or writing practice or a meditation practice or a cooking practice.

Over the past couple of years, more and more of my practice is accepting things that are outside of my control. You have to have faith and to give it up. I don't mean faith in a god or faith in an icon. I mean you have to have faith that there's some guiding principle that's greater than yourself that helps to achieve good. In order to go on, you have to have faith that there's a little more good. There's some guiding principle that will edge you toward benevolent.

In quantum physics, there's the idea of the wave and the particle. The benefits of contemplation practices are that you begin to get more waves than particles. It's not that waves are good and particles are bad. Think of it this way, waves have a way of going through you. A particle gets lodged. It either gets lodged as a memory, or trauma or a habit and then the particle spins in your being. What we're trying to do in all of these practices, and in writing, is watch the particles but allow them to become waves, or wavelike.

The stories we tell are the particles. They're not bad, but they are the story making part. The waves allow you not to hold on to them.

Be Your Own Sweetheart

We cannot connect to others until we connect to ourselves.

A natural outcome of developing a relationship with a spirit who lovingly listens and holds your story is you learn to connect deeply to and love yourself. We cannot connect to others until we connect to ourselves and all parts of the stories we're holding. We then begin to experience deep empathy with ourselves.

Write it!

List five nice things you can do for yourself today.

Anything Is Inspiration

Anything you see that you touch, or taste or smell has the ability to be inspiration. If you're walking and the smell of figs is so pungent, that can serve as inspiration for a story. Anything can be an inspiration, it's what attaches to the moment of inspiration. How does the smell of figs attach to something else that inspires you? Then you string it along to make a story, to create an idea.

—Brette Popper

I have a friend who looks at her computer as a form of spirit. "How could it not be?" she asks. "It's my portal to connection and others."

You can make anything sacred. Bedazzle your life. Imbue your technology with the same qualities as your inner guide; let it too be a vessel. Create a halo around you and your story, including your writing technology.

Write it!

Describe your halo.

You Are Enough

There are no missing pieces.

One of my favorite books growing up was Shel Silverstein's *The Missing Piece*. My father used to read it to me every night. The book centers around an individual who thinks they're missing something, and they're going out into the world to find the piece that will complete them. One after another, each piece they find is not quite right. Some are too small, others too big. Some are too shy, others too flashy. At a certain point, they think they've found their match, and oh, what a blissful, albeit short, union they share—until one of them grows, and they no longer fit. Each potential partner has something to offer, but nothing quite lasts.

Ultimately the piece realizes they're not missing anything. They just need to learn how to roll on their own.

Write it!

Write about a time you made do with what you had, and it was enough.

Story Architect

Julia Sedlock is a writer, designer, and community advocate based in the Hudson Valley. Her first book, *Creatures Are Stirring: A Guide to Architectural Companionship*, coauthored with Joseph Altshuler, was released by Applied Research and Design in 2022.

Architects begin every project by asking how our proposal will sit in relationship to the other structures, people and landscapes around it. We present possibilities for how different sets of people might engage in different kinds of activities across space and time. We either minimize interaction by placing walls that separate one space or person from another, or facilitate interaction with halls and windows that physically or visually connect them. We also create moods and atmospheres that impact how people might feel in a given space and time. Using form, materiality, texture, color, lighting and acoustics, architects can design a space to feel upbeat and energizing, or somber and calming. We start with a vague sketch, an intention, an intuition or a hypothesis, and build complexity through rounds of rigorous experimentation to test if the specificity of our design solution will achieve the intended effect.

Architects don't wander over to a plot and start piling materials on top of each other and hope for the best. They don't do this at all. They dream and imagine, envision, and then sketch and sketch, plot and plan. The same is true for us, except instead of building buildings, we're building connection and relationships through storytelling.

Imagine your story structure. What does yours look like? What is the foundation? Scaffolding? How many stories? How many rooms? How does your story create an atmosphere?

Write it!

What is the plan for your story? You can use words or draw.

Release

Take a deep breath in. On the out breath, flutter your lips like a horse.
Repeat three times.

How You Do Anything Is
How You Do Everything

Mindfulness is your personalized practice of coming into the present moment with awareness, attention, and care.

Mindfulness doesn't have to happen in a yoga or meditation studio or with a special app or teacher. It's something that happens as you move through your day. It can change, mutate, grow, shrink, slow down, and speed up. It also comes in small caring actions we take.

Notice how you are reading this book right now. Are you comfortable? Are you breathing with ease? Are you thirsty? Hungry? Rushed? Distracted? Are you cold? Hot? Write about what you are noticing about yourself in this moment.

You are doing a mindfulness practice right now.

Only Things You Love

Carla Zanoni is an Argentine American writer, poet, and digital media expert who was the first Latina named to the *Wall Street Journal*'s masthead; she is the first audience development strategy leader at TED.

There has to be a foundation of practice. It's a practice of showing up at your seat. The same as a meditation cushion or sitting before an altar. In many ways, my desk is an altar. I have special stones, a singing bowl and all these kinds of things in front of me. It's creating a space and showing up in a space. And dedicating time and space to listening to myself, trusting myself and my process to just let it be. In that process I start hearing things that can only be explained as messages or prompts or a guiding hand from what I believe is my higher power. My higher power can be explained in many ways, but one important way is that it's an energy that's within me and outside of me that's a support and makes me feel safe even when things feel turbulent and maybe really emotional and feel like they're not things I can control. Just a guiding hand.

So, it's really important to me that my desk only has things on it that I love. Everything in front of me needs to be incredibly beautiful. I have special stones that have meaning to me. Sometimes when writing, I'll grab one that has meaning to me in my hand so there's a tactile experience. A beautiful broken seashell, a friendship stone someone gave to me, a beautiful candle. I don't think you have to be particularly witchy, it's just about things that can make you feel present and inspired;

things that remind you that there is beauty in the world. Beauty can be a way to connect with something larger than yourself and become a conduit to bring that into the world through writing.

Write it!

Describe your writing altar.

Lose Your Balance

I am rooted, but I flow.
—Virginia Woolf[17]

Sometimes the best way to find your center is to shift away from that center slightly, or even a lot. You only really know what balance feels like when you move between being off balance and then finding your way back. Mindfulness is not about seeking perfection and constant serenity; it's instead the practice of becoming aware of when you're on and off the beam and adjusting as you go.

Your body naturally wants to release feelings, sensations, and attachments that are not benefiting you. We can feel this as we are breathing. Our breath can tell us when we are at ease and when we are not, and conversely with our breath, we can influence how we feel. Our breathing is one of the only bodily functions that can be either automatic or voluntary (up to a point).

You may not have a highwire handy to work with balance and trust, but you have your body and access to the floor, a wall, or a chair. In whatever way is comfortable to you, move off balance—blinking one eye, shifting your weight, or actually balancing on one leg, if this is possible and safe for you.

Notice what changes and what remains the same.

Write it!

What does it feel like to move away from and return to balance?

Turn Straw into Gold

The most humiliating thing that ever happened
to you is the medicine someone else needs.

Before Facebook and Instagram, there was a project called PostSecret;
it began with pop-up live events. The creator, Frank Warren, invited
people to the event, and on arrival everyone was invited to share a
secret on a Post-it, something they had never told anyone, and then
they stuck their secret on the wall. Invariably, there would be some
recurring themes, some surprises, and a big range of the quality and
severity of the secret shared. What was often the case is that people
felt better after unburdening themselves as a result of releasing
something they were holding—and they felt better knowing everyone else has secrets too.

We keep secrets for a variety of reasons, ranging from shame,
guilt, and fear to mild embarrassment. For most of us, the conceal-
ment is more punishing than the secret itself. It's as if we are blocking our bodies' natural digestion of the material, like an emotional
constipation of sorts. Our culture can reenforce some of these behaviors with hateful and limiting policies, like "don't ask, don't tell,"
where people are led to conclude it's safer to keep a secret than to
share it.

You have the power to transform your difficult experiences into
strength by sharing them and allowing them to make their way to
someone who needs to hear your message (and that person could be
you).

Name a secret you have never shared and make a list of reasons that you are not sharing it.

Write down a humiliating experience—you don't need to share it—and turn straw to gold.

Heartbeats

A book is a heart that only beats in the chest of another.
—Rebecca Solnit[18]

The second you open a book, you're involved in an intimate, private conversation. No other art form is quite this way. It is solitary, private, elusive, and secretive. The delight and pleasure of the story is just for you. Reading offers a private communication between you and the author, who you at once feel intimately connected to and most likely have no relationship with at all.

Reading is the act of taking in someone else's story, without also taking in a body. It's almost like a long-distance relationship—it offers intimacy, but you choose how frequently you engage, which can be easier on a sensitive nervous system. You can read in many forms—via audiobook or podcast, online or in print, being read to or reading aloud to yourself. The healing is that you're taking in someone else's story that they spent time putting together. This transmission can be transformative on its own.

Reading is here to support you. It's an ever-available, all-encompassing, reliable way to open up all the windows and doors while holding on to someone's hand—that's yours and yours alone—to provide comfort, enjoyment, connection, and nourishment.

Try it!

Read for twenty minutes.

Let Go More

It's always an option to let go more.

If, right now, you are having any thoughts, emotions, or sensations that you are actually aware of that are hindering you, bring them to mind right now.

On an inhale, say silently to yourself, *Let*.

On an exhale say silently to yourself, *Go*.

Inhale *Let*.

Exhale *Go*.

Continue for one minute. As you repeat the phrase, invite in any energies or ideas that you're aware of that you would like to let go of. What is holding you back from sharing what you need to share? It's always an option to let go more.

Write it!

What is something or someone you are holding on to?

PART FIVE

Connect

UNFURL

I arrive at the lofted coffee shop in downtown Manhattan the same way I do for most meetings: breathless, determined, and detached. I am cloaked in a full suit of armor, with hair pulled back into a sleek French twist, fitted black leather jacket zipped up to the collar, tote bag equipped with two black pens, and a black notebook; I am primed to present my professional arsenal to a new client.

———

When my mentor Jillian Pransky asks to meet with me outside of class, I instantly spin a story in my head about what she'll want to talk about. I know she's working on a book, and with my background in publishing, I am prepared to offer advice (solicited or not) and guidance on the publishing process. This mantra was running through my head: *I have the experience you need.*

I hope she will hire me to amplify her story.

Jillian is seated in the far back corner and greets me with a wide, warm expression and soft eyes. Natural light from above pools around her. Draped in a loose knitted beige off-the-shoulder sweater, she wears a different kind of uniform, a stillness that startles me. In class she teaches that yoga practice is a deep well of self-love and acceptance and offers tools to listen to ourselves, to others, and to the conditions of our environment, but I have never seen it embodied like this outside of the yoga studio. I didn't realize that attitude, that presence, can walk around in the real world with the rest of us.

I take a seat but leave my jacket on. I have barely started my pitch when she interrupts me by taking a slow breath in and out. Looking me in the eye, she says casually, "I need to know your story." This jars me like an unexpected speed bump.

I have no idea what she is talking about. She already knows my professional background. I remind myself *I have the experience you need* and breathe into the armor, still zipped up tight around my chest. I take a shallow breath and catch the smokey smell of coffee around us and respond, "My story?"

"Your story." She nods. "I like to know the stories of people before I work with them."

"All right." I clear the suspicion from my throat and follow up more softly, "How much do you want to know?"

"Why don't you just start at the beginning and keep going from there."

I take a deep breath and feel leather pushing against my ribs. *Do I know how to do that?* I have spent most of my life avoiding what Jillian is asking of me. I prefer to parcel out, compartmentalize, tie up, and mute different parts of my story; I present the versions of myself I think other people want. But this time something is different. By this point in our relationship, I have clocked hundreds of hours learning to trust Jillian in the yoga studio, where she guides me into relaxation and a state of wholeness. The restorative postures that Jillian teaches are often vulnerable; many involve lying propped up by bolsters and blocks on the ground with my heart and belly exposed. Her teachings offer ways to safely surrender to vulnerability and adjust with props as needed. As I sit, to my surprise, I feel just as safe in the coffee shop. I am talking to someone who has already seen all of me—there is nothing to hide.

I am still hesitant to allow my yoga-self to crash my business meeting. But before my ego brain can intervene with the curated script that lives in my forehead, I feel my center of gravity drop down into my throat, then my chest, then my gut, where my true voice lives. I find new words.

I talk unfiltered for a long time, like an endless exhale. I breeze and bubble through the landscape of my childhood: my vibrant, chaotic, and loving family; the dozen or so moves before I turned eighteen; my complicated relationship with my mother. Jillian nods.

I don't know what to say when I begin to describe college. I hit another speed bump. I normally detour around this time period, including the suicidal depression and medical leave that resulted. Yet there is something about Jillian's presence that guides me to slow down. I don't skip over and camouflage with a joke. Instead, I tell her how in college I lived a double life. From the outside I appeared to be thriving, but slowly, and then quickly, my moods sank so low, it was impossible to keep up. "In a matter of weeks," I say, "I lost the desire to leave my dorm room and, eventually, the will to live."

I intend to stop there, but Jillian's gentle, receptive gaze set me at ease, so I continue. I share that I had been visited by campus police and put on a suicide watch. I feel dizzy. I usually keep this zipped up. But in that café, in the presence of my teacher and friend, I give voice to the bits of my story I normally silence. I breathe in steadiness from her quiet support, and I breathe out my truth. To my shock, she doesn't seem surprised or disappointed. She offers instead an open, nonjudgmental container, and my words pour into it like a waterfall.

For years well-meaning people in my life had told me to keep this experience to myself—they warned no one would hire me, date me, marry me, if they knew this secret—and my experience transformed from pain to silence to shame. I built up thick walls and never let anyone truly hear or know me, including myself. Over time, this pretending and hiding caused a different and deeper harm than the original depression itself.

I'm flooded with memories of what it had been like to share my story in the past. In my memory I'm always outnumbered by doctors and being evaluated. I'm asked to rate myself. There's a right answer and a wrong answer. I try to outmaneuver them and bring my own clipboard. I sit upright, like them, and take notes, like them. Over time, I learn to confine and punish the story—my story—itself. This pattern repeats itself when I am with friends, family, and boyfriends.

In those cases, I learn to tell my story like a badge of honor or rite of passage. I make myself the butt of my own jokes.

This is my first time sharing these parts of my story with a peer who is nonjudgmental, relaxed, unrushed, and caring, not because they weren't around—there have always been plenty of people who love me and care about me—but because I wouldn't allow myself the risk. It felt safer to lock myself up and use my body as a shield.

Sharing with Jillian is like waking up from a dream state. The story I am telling is from fifteen years ago, but for a moment, it feels like I am describing events from the day before. I pause and look around the room, intuitively tracking my environment to steady myself. I notice light wood columns, white walls. I hear lively conversations, spoons knocking against porcelain crockery, and steam whistling at the espresso bar. I feel the hard wooden chair beneath me.

Connecting with my senses grounds me and brings me back to the moment I am in, safe and whole. I soften my shoulders. I notice the texture of my shirt on my skin, the air circulating in the room. As if readying for a meditation, I close my eyes for a moment.

I open my eyes a few seconds later. She is still here, still calm; nothing has changed. "Hi," she says.

Her eyes tell me she is in no rush, which helps me slow down. Unconsciously, I begin mirroring her body language and posture. I start to feel more embodied, relaxed, and trusting. I wonder if there is no right or wrong way to tell to my story, just what it is. It's mine.

As I continue, my voice sounds different to my ears—rounder and warmer, more like a singing bowl than a siren. I feel transported to certain resting yoga postures, like *supta baddha konasana*, a reclined yoga posture where the legs are supported and the chest—and heart—peel open in a gesture of receptivity and trust.

I shed the armor I arrived with. I am no longer resizing, filtering, and targeting the words to fit what I think she wants to hear or what will get me where I think I want to go. Instead, I release the story that is ready to be heard: of my wounded twenty-year-old self, isolated and scared, vulnerable and unwell. I didn't even know I had been dragging her around everywhere I went.

I feel a fleeting sensation, a prick.

When I am done talking, I look up. I inhale, stunned. I had totally forgotten I was trying to get a job.

"Lisa," she says, "thank you."

She takes a breath, as if to sweep clean the air between us. "Y'know, you never really have to tell your whole story like that again." Observing my creased brow, she answers my unspoken question: "I never tell my whole story when I'm teaching," she says. "You'll learn how to tell bits and pieces of it and use it as a tool. You will help people with it, like you've helped me just now."

I find this comforting, like a promise I didn't know I was seeking. She offers space, the gift of being a witness, and helps me loosen the tight bow I have tied around my trauma. I look around the table and now feel three of us sitting there: me, Jillian, and my twenty-year-old self. I see her long brown hair, her tight olive skin. I see a beauty mark on her cheek I hadn't noticed before. Looking closely, yes, I can see some sadness, and I also see how beautiful and strong she is. She is fully grown. She isn't so broken and doesn't need me to protect her anymore.

As if on cue, the waiter arrives with the check. As we pull out our wallets, I watch my younger self stand up to leave the table. She throws her jacket over her shoulder and walks away, free to leave. I know she will come back when she needs me, or when I need her. But for now, she has been heard and has places to go.

Contemplate it!

What happens to a story when it's held in love?

Trusting Relationships Heal

Beyond any technique, relationships are what heal.
—Dr. Lewis Mehl Madrona[19]

Studies have shown that trusting relationships can help heal trauma by establishing safety; extinguishing shame; soothing stress; integrating compartmentalized parts; decreasing feelings of hopelessness and isolation; letting go of the past and making room for a new story; feeling heard and seen; and reflecting and finding feelings of inspiration, joy, and connection.

No matter how hard you try, you can't transform yourself by yourself—you're just not that powerful. It takes an outside source, perspective, and energy, the same way pollen left alone can't fertilize other flowers; it needs to be moved around by bees, wind, or another creature. In my experience, this transformation begins with trusting one person with your story. My story about my mental health crisis in college, which had been buried for years, bloomed into something unrecognizable when I shared it with a loving, nonjudgmental listener. Part of it was the connection it forged between us, but the more powerful part was the model of how to hold my own vulnerable story with love. As a result of that conversation, I learned how to hold compassionate space in a whole new way, which transformed every aspect of my storytelling experience.

In taking this next step, it's important to pause. *It's crucial to choose this person carefully.* This person can even be you, perhaps in your journal, or prayer with your higher power. Next you can move outward to a good listener—a friend, a therapist, a doctor, a healer, a spiritual guide, a coach, a mentor, or a teacher. What's important is that you *choose* this person, that they are someone who feels safe, grounded, and trustworthy to you. Your story can only grow and benefit in the presence of a regulated person. If you don't already have someone like this, I'll walk you through ways to seek them out. They are out there. I promise.

In our culture we're often skipping this critical stage of trusting one person—a stage your nervous system needs in order to heal, transform, and ultimately share effectively and critically on a group level. Instead, we are often instructed to *go big or go home*. We seek followers, fame, impact, and results over intimate trusting connection. The true meaning of our stories is revealed to us once we share them with someone we trust.

Contemplate it!

Take a moment to reflect on a time you shared and wished you hadn't. Now, reflect on a time you shared and found that it helped.

Sharing and Recovery

Sharing and listening is a two-way street. There are a few reasons why it's important to start sharing your story with one chosen person. One-on-one healing is the cornerstone of all Western healing dating back to Greco-Roman times and the foundation of all healing and transforming relationships. This is also true for shamanic traditions, healing arts, and the way we conceive of primary relationships in our social constructs, like parent-child, partner-partner, friend-friend, teacher-student, doctor-patient, or editor-writer and writer-reader for example.

One-on-one is the most efficient way to grow and connect. On a physical level, we are better able to soak up the security from one body when we are in private company, simply because there are no other distractions or obstacles. This is why most therapists, as well as healing-arts practitioners, doctors, nurses, and healers of all stripes generally offer private consultations.

This relationship is the basis for moving beyond your story and the confines of your own lived experience. As you release stories, verbally or not, to a secure person whom you trust, you can release yourself from the limits of your own lived experience and begin to turn the page and rewrite your story.

There are a few frameworks to help deepen our understanding of this connection. From a scientific lens, there has been important new research that shows that when a story is held with love, it can play a critical role in healing trauma. As Dr. James Gordon writes in *The Transformation*, "In sharing ourselves and our stories, we're also overcoming the fear of judgment, the pride and the shame that have fed the isolation bred by trauma."[20]

Listening and the Nervous System

Before a word is even uttered, the nervous system is already communicating—we scan our surroundings to pick up messages on whether the bodies around us are safe or threatening, whether they will lead us toward danger or toward thriving. We tell a story by how we are breathing, how we are holding our bodies, whether we are giving off an open-minded or close-minded energy, whether our eyes are soft or hard, whether our muscles are tense or relaxed. Think back to some of the listening cues we discussed in Part One; these were designed to give embodied signals to the speaker that our bodies are listening.

We can sense whether someone is in a heightened fight-or-flight response or rest-and-digest by observing the visible tension in their body, rate of breath, smell, gaze, and a host of other cues. We need to be relaxed and at ease to receive these messages accurately; otherwise we misread the signs. This is true for the safety of the body, the safety of our precious stories, and the safety of our emotional, creative, and spiritual lives.

When we are relaxed and regulated, we are able to establish a connection with one person; we also experience a sense of understanding and confidence and are naturally able to lift our voices into the world. This connection itself serves as a form of relaxation. It's like a turbo-restorative yoga pose or meditation practice. When we attune ourselves to a relaxed nervous system, we can literally borrow from it to ground and orient our own nervous system. This is always important in establishing secure relationships and confidence but is especially so when you are triggered by a trauma response. A person we trust makes us feel heard and seen; we don't have to utter a word for this kind of exchange to take place. Our bodies tell stories through our nervous systems all the time. Once you have established this safety with the person you are talking to, your nervous system is not only wired to find security and safety but also to find connection and understanding and to seek sameness with everyone else. So when we create this connection with someone, we will be able to share our truth and feel seen and heard, which emboldens us to take risks, find joy, and experience deeper and more nuanced emotions.

Since our nervous system is a two-way street, we also share these qualities with others when we are regulated—making the world a safer place for everyone in our vicinity, regardless of whether verbal storytelling is happening between you (more on this later). You become a safe receptacle for others to share their stories too. Of course, the opposite is also true, and when we feel unsafe and threatened, we give off that message through our bodies and impact the bodies around us.

Whole-Body Storytelling

Whole-body storytelling is biological and psychological and can be understood as a form of trauma healing. In recent years, trauma specialists have developed a field of study called polyvagal theory

(PVT), which describes how we communicate through our nervous systems to establish safety and connection with each other. Developed in 1994 by Stephen Porges, PVT has expanded over the subsequent decades, leading trauma therapists across the globe to adopt this new understanding of how embodiment practices offer healing from trauma. Porges writes, "To fulfill our biological imperative of connectedness, our personal agenda needs to be directed toward making individuals feel safe."[21]

PVT-trained therapists use various cues and activities rooted in either playful response or restorative practices to dynamically shift the client's nervous system. What this shows is that a dynamic relationship, similar to what we experience when we are entrusting someone with our story, can shift nervous systems to rest and restore. While not exactly the same, this offering is reminiscent of what I experienced when I shared my story with Jillian and what you also may experience when you share a vulnerable story with a trusted other. The sharing of the vulnerable story itself can aid in shifting away from hyperarousal or a fight, flight, freeze, or fawn state and into a relaxation response, where you can become receptive to understanding and being understood. While PVT experts are focusing on trauma recovery, this research is useful for all kinds of storytelling. The embodiment practices developed from PVT are reminiscent of mindfulness practices, like restorative yoga and meditation—except instead of using props and breath to relax and move from a reactive state into rest and restore, in PVT we use each other's nervous systems.

Open Your Heart

Whole-body listening and connecting begins with a connection to the heart. When our voices, spirits, and actions are aligned, we are primed to form healing connections. The sharing can happen in big and small ways—from a friendly exchange to speaking your truth, standing up for something you believe in, releasing tender trauma stories, or simply sharing space and letting your body tell the story with a sigh, a smile, or a tear. The first step is sharing with one trusted and understanding person. When you are regulated, you will intuitively know who to share what with. And you will intuitively know when to listen and when to be quiet.

Our heart is not a revolving door; it is sacred, tender, and emotional. Our heart is also not a metaphor; it's a vital organ, protected by a cage of ribs and pillows of lungs. We can choose whether to make our heart available.

One way to ready yourself for sharing is to open the heart. Even a little bit of a heart opening through movement can have a profound impact. I'll offer a few practices to try. Be gentle with yourself with these practices. If any make you feel nervous or unsafe in any way, please don't do them. Some are better for different times and for different environments. There is nothing to gain by forcing, fixing, or pushing yourself here.

Try it!

Heart Tapping

Lightly tap the skin over your heart area (along your breastbone) with your fingers to say hello to your heart center. Take a few rounds of deep breaths, in and out. What do you feel? What don't you feel?

This subtle practice that you can pull out anywhere is a gentle reminder to connect within before connecting outside.

Heart Opening

If you are in a private space and would like a more full-bodied experience, try this. This one requires some props; you can use a pillow, rolled-up blanket or towel, or a yoga bolster, if you have one. To set up, find a clearing on the floor that looks inviting, a bed, or a patch of grass. Place your pillow, blanket, or bolster on the ground and then lie down on your back on top of it, placing whatever you choose right under your lower ribs, or where a bra strap might go. Lie down with your legs extended or bent and breathe here for one minute. You can modify how intense this backbend is by placing a pillow under your head.

Heart Expanding

Here's a practice for anyone looking for a more active expression. If you have any shoulder or wrist pain or limitation, skip over this one.

Standing, interlace your fingers behind your lower back (you can also hold on to a towel or belt) and stretch them away from your shoulders. Inhale, lifting your heart toward the sky, and exhale, stretching your hands toward the ground. Switch the interlace of your hands and repeat.

Write it!

What does your heart feel?

Only Speak If It Improves the Silence

A loving silence often has far more power to heal and to connect than the most well-intentioned words.

—Rachel Naomi Remen[22]

It's important to say what we need to say, and it's often more important to know what *not* to say—in other words, what to leave out. It's a way of giving space and oxygen to our stories and those around us. Read between the lines. Step into the silence and into the exhale of each sentence. Even the stories that aren't uttered out loud still take up space. They are like ether; they are the space between what's uttered, which gives us meaning.

Before you speak, ask yourself:

Does it need to be said?
Does it need to be said by you?
Does it need to be said now?
Is it kind?

Healthy Boundaries Support Connection and Joy

Pause before sharing a personal trauma and ask:
Are you sharing to be of service, ask yourself if it really is of service.
Are you processed enough, are you self-aware enough and
will the audience really be able to hear?
Is it your turn to speak, are you making space for anyone more
vulnerable than you?
—Laura Khoudari, pioneer in trauma-informed
strength training, writer, speaker, wellness coach,
and author of the book *Lifting Heavy Things:*
Healing Trauma One Rep at a Time

What we take in, what we listen to, impacts us on emotional, biological, and creative levels. There are times when it's best not to listen fully. Not every story exists for our greater good. This is certainly the case when encountering stories based in hate, violence, falsehoods, or ignorance, or when we're emotionally triggered in any way. This is also true of text messages, emails, and any other communication. Not every question is a command. It's always an option not to respond.

The good news is that we have tools for how we choose to take stories in. We have a lot of filters to help us with this digitally, energetically, and emotionally. You can become more aware of how stories are impacting your body as you take them in.

Here is some everyday, practical, and tactical guidance. What are your communication habits? Our addiction to technology, to our smartphones, email, social media, and video games, is more pervasive and arguably more dangerous than our addiction to drugs and alcohol. We can do something about this. It begins with awareness. Check your own behavior and explore the following ways of filtering how information comes your way. This isn't meant to be punishing as much as suggestive. Scan below and see which, if any, of these options feels worthwhile.

Suggested Practice (Choose Two to Start!):

Count to ten before replying to an email or text.

Begin the day with natural light.

Avoid screens the first and last twenty minutes of the day.

Schedule uninterruptable time in your week.

Create email folders to filter information as it comes in.

Don't send emails before 8:00 a.m. or after 8:00 p.m.

Count to three before responding.

Close your eyes.

Meditate by focusing on a sound or vibration.

Turn off your phone.

Name any that I missed.

On How We Tell Our Stories Matters

Elizabeth L. Silver is a novelist, lawyer, and the author of the forthcoming novel *The Majority*. She also wrote *The Execution of Noa P. Singleton* and the memoir *The Tincture of Time: A Memoir of (Medical) Uncertainty*. She is the founder and director of Onward Literary Mentoring and lives in Los Angeles with her family.

With respect to legal situations and high crisis situations and any sort of interpersonal relationships—how you say it, what you say and when you say it matters. If you wait too long to apologize or you wait too long to say something there's a statute of limitations that's legal and also personal, right? Some people might say, "Oh, you waited too long to apologize," or "you waited too long to say that thing." And also, if how you say it doesn't match the language that's also confusing to the recipient. How we tell our stories is essential to their effectiveness.

How you say that story and specifically what you are saying—and I feel like I do this all the time, I might be talking to someone and think, Oh, I put my foot in my mouth; I didn't need to give away all those details. They didn't need to know all the details about my morning breakfast, they just needed to hear what time I got to work. And instead, I told them all about how my blender broke and then I had to go out and buy bananas . . . we'll go through a whole narrative that matters to us, but that's not necessarily relevant for the outcome or for that reason. So, when we think about this in law, we think what are the relevant details that this person who's going to make a decision about you, what do they need to know? And the individuals who are telling that, don't always know that because they're not trained lawyers. The same is true when you're writing a story, whether it's fiction or nonfiction. It's the idea of writing to find the story. We've all done this when you write 100 pages to get to the first one. Or you write many paragraphs to get to the first one, and you're often starting on page 20. When we're talking and telling our stories we don't always know how to do that because it doesn't come naturally. In our heads we think we need to explain.

Write it!

Write about . . .

* a time telling your story offered protection for you.
* a time telling your story offered protection for someone else.
* a time your story *could* have offered protection, but you stayed silent.

It Is Through Words That We Find Each Other

Write a letter to begin sharing.

I've always been an avid letter writer. I love writing love letters, thank-you letters, fan letters, and birthday cards. I love pen pals, sliding notes under the door, leaving Post-its in suitcases and backpacks to be found later. To me, there are few greater pleasures than sealing an envelope and sending it off. I love the mystery of it, the romance, the hopefulness, and the secrecy. A letter is like a sloweddown conversation. One slow breath and then another.

Electronic boundaries and old-fashioned technologies are friends to your nervous system in this context. They are a way to pause and let others in at the same time, a powerful first step toward connection, whether you send anything or not. You can consider letter writing a trauma-informed writing practice.

Write it!

Choose a prompt (or two or three) that inspires you and write the following:

a fan letter to someone you admire
a secret admirer letter
a letter asking for advice
a letter to file a complaint
a letter to your neighbor
a letter to a body part

an "I miss you" letter
a just-because letter
a "this reminded me of you" letter
a letter to the future
a letter to the past
a letter to your favorite food
a letter to someone you lost
a letter to an animal friend
a letter to a favorite character in a book
a letter to . . . (fill in the blank)

Then, send it.

Guide to Finding a Listener

We can create safety for ourselves by
surrounding ourselves with safe bodies.

We don't all have intact and reliable support systems.

Frequently when I teach, students will ask me how to find a safe person or how to know if their person is the right kind of safe. It can be hard to establish safety, especially if you've been burned by someone you trust or if you're working with trauma. Begin by grounding yourself with any of the practices I shared earlier or others you know.

We are constantly emitting signs to each other that indicate whether we are safe or not. Here are some cues: look for a regular breathing pattern, relaxed muscles, and open demeanor. You will know the cues that matter to you. You will feel it in your body, in your gut, in the hairs at the back of your neck. Your inner GPS will tell you.

Trust your breath. Trust your belly and your back and how you feel around this person. Do you feel relaxed? At ease? Content?

Try it!

Choose someone who makes you feel comfortable, safe, relaxed, supported, and accepted. Make a list of what that means for you.
Choose someone who brings out the best in you.
Choose a "yes" person in your life, someone who reflects back what is good, what is working, what inspires, and what delights.
Choose someone who opens doors and makes you see things in a new way.
Choose someone who lifts you up and gives you energy.

Choose someone who reminds you of your own intention and basic goodness and worth.

Choose someone who makes you feel brilliant, loved—like you can do anything.

Write it!

Describe your ideal trusted listener, whether this is someone imagined or real. Make a list of their character traits. If anyone comes to mind, name them. Otherwise, write down the characteristics of your ideal person and begin with that ideal list.

On Entering the Story

Lewis Mehl Madrona, MD, is the author of *Coyote Medicine*, *Coyote Healing*, *Coyote Wisdom*, *Narrative Medicine*, *Healing the Mind Through the Power of Story*, and his most recent book, with Barbara Mainguy, *Remapping Your Mind*.

I've realized that indigenous is everywhere. I am thinking about one of my favorite narrative therapists, Ibn-Sina who practiced in Persia in the tenth century. My favorite story that I tell pretty often is when he was treating a young man who thought he was a cow and was refusing to eat. He goes to see this young man, and of course the Sultan, the father of this young man is distressed because his son, this young man wants to be sacrificed and cooked and fed to the people. So, Ibn-Sina came to see him and looked him up and down and said, "I don't know, Mr. prince, you're scrawny looking, I don't know how we could even get one meal out of you. I think we have to fatten you up before taking you to the slaughterhouse." So, the prince agreed, that was a plan. So, Ibn-Sina came to visit him every day and the prince improved. One day the prince said to Ibn-Sina, "You know it's really hard for me to break the news to you and I really don't want to upset you, but it turns out I'm not a cow."

We try to follow Ibn-Sina's example of entering the story. We're too quick to give advice. When you enter into people's stories it means you have to listen to their story for quite a while to see how things work. One of the things that I do with everyone I see clinically, is to get a life story. There are medical questions that are required for billing but beyond that I try to get their life story, how they see their lives, what are the major periods of their lives as they see them. What are the high points and the low points and the turning points? How do they explain things? This is a question I often ask people.

Invite people to listen to the whole story and let go of the idea that they need to fix it, correct it. If you keep listening, you will find, you will be given ideas of how to interact with somebody.

Fire the Coach

Listen inward. Are there any voices in your head that aren't yours?

For years, a typical day for me looked something like this: I dragged myself out of bed wearing a layer of shame about the past and a fear of the future. The first thing I reached for was a coffee the size of my torso. I forced myself to do something uncomfortable first, like run for forty-five minutes along the West Side Highway at 6:30 a.m. I even invited an imaginary coach in sweats to come along. After my run was over, she stayed with me all day long, blowing a whistle and scream-ing shaming remarks disguised as affirmations, like, "You can do it!" or "Be the boss!" to the tune of the *Rocky* soundtrack or a Beyoncé empowerment anthem. Sometimes the whistle would get louder and sometimes the voice would get meaner; she might snarl, "What's wrong with you!?" if I started to flag in my sprint through life.

Rest wasn't an option. Growing up the child of a baby-booming, glass-ceiling-breaking, immigrant overachiever, I was raised to acknowledge how lucky I was to have the opportunities I had and to never take them for granted. This served me well in some ways: I got good grades. I did well in sports. But I didn't know how to stop or slow down. I was told I was wasting my life if I took a sick day from school. So, early on, I, like many others, oriented my day around pleasing and keeping up with that internal (and even real-life) coach telling me to strive, push, and try even harder. This coach spoke to me in different voices, sometimes using my parents' voices, my bosses' voices, my teachers' voices, and my friends' voices until ulti-mately, she disguised herself in my voice. I didn't know how to listen to my own voice, because I could barely hear myself amid all the shouting in my head.

What I learned was that the best way to stop a harmful voice was to replace it with something else. So I chased rest with the same fervor that I had chased my previous ambition. I logged hundreds of hours in restorative yoga teacher trainings. I read all the books on rest and relaxation I could. I took yoga nidra, restorative yoga, and gasped at the statistics around sleep deprivation and stress. Over time resting became a habit and a cornerstone of my day—and a new voice in my head.

Try it!

Is anyone yelling at you, telling you to improve, fix, tighten, or push? Is there a coach inside of you masquerading as your own voice?
Mute them.

Write it!

Now, imagine your *ideal* coach. Imagine someone (or thing) who makes you feel good, supported, loved, happy, and inspired. Imagine a coach who wants you to be comfortable and relaxed. Describe them. Describe their energy, what they look like and sound like. Give them a name and invite them along with you during the day.

Rest

Offer yourself what you need.

Take a moment to relax your eyes. Here are a few options to consider. You can close your eyes, and beneath your eyelids slowly look side to side, up and down, in circular motions going clockwise and counterclockwise. You might also try cupping your palms over your eyes and soaking up the nourishment of your own shadow and your own energy. You might apply a little pressure and massage around the eyes or simply take a break from the screen. Or choose any other method that you know works well for you.

Listening, a Peak Pose

When we make space to listen to our own
stories, we also make space to hear others'.

How we position our bodies matters. The shapes, or postures, we
assume when we listen impact *how* we listen. How we hold our bodies also signals that capacity to our peers, both people who we are
directing our attention to and those in our general environment. The
way we hold ourselves echoes into the space around us. It ripples out.

Often in a yoga class, an experienced teacher will design postures
that prepare the body for what's called a "peak pose." For our purposes, let's consider listening to be our peak pose and build a practice
for ideal listening.

There are a number of ways to help the body relax and release;
here are a few quick practices you can pull out at a moment's notice.
In these exercises we are slowing down time in some ways so we can
better set ourselves up for peaceful and creative reactions to what's
around us. This will both help with conflict resolution and increase
our creative output and general sense of well-being.

Try it!

1. Assess your surroundings. Become aware of your conditions—
    the sounds, smells, and beings around you and how they make
    you feel. Notice the weather and temperature. Notice whether
    you need to make any adjustments in your position to feel more
    comfortable and at ease. If this is not possible, then listening is
    not possible. Full stop. You'll need to alter your environment in
    some way or try another time.

2. Find a comfortable seat. Pause and take a few breaths and check again. Do you need to make any modifications? Note the nearest door and window. Notice the weather.
3. Focus. Once you feel secure, take a moment to plant your feet on the ground and place your hands somewhere that feels good to you—maybe your lap or gently on a surface. Avoid crossing your arms and covering your throat, heart, and lungs. That is your primary listening and communication channel. Keeping them open will signify to your partner that you're available to listen. Again, reconfirm with yourself that you feel safe in this position.
4. Check your breathing. Are you breathing fully?
5. Prime yourself to receive.
6. Receive. When you are listening, let the speaker know you are listening. If it feels authentic, place your hands to your heart to express empathy. Options include nodding, placing a hand on the heart, making eye contact, snapping, bringing your palms together, smiling, or anything else that feels right to you.
7. Avoid interrupting or asking for more information. Only take in what is being offered.
8. Listen for what you identify with, for what you love.

Now these may seem like a lot of steps, but they'll get easier as you become more accustomed to this practice. When you find yourself in a more challenging situation, my hope is that you will lean into one of these practices—maybe it's a breath cue, or a sound meditation, a quick note to center yourself and align your nervous system. You will be able to meet the moment with the required awareness and openness to connect with the best possible outcome for all. You become a natural part of an environment that makes listening possible. Your presence alone is the power others need to speak their truths.

The Alchemy of Listening

Sharing can be a form of transformation. The
meaning of the story itself may change.

For many people, a story changes—in intention, cadence, and
meaning—when they share it live with someone they sense is listening. It changes even more if you share it with someone you trust.

This phenomenon is not just a felt sense; it's also a biological phenomenon. When the speaker feels as if their story is being held by a
trustworthy body and when the listening body is listening wholeheartedly, it triggers biochemical changes in the brain that cause us
to open up and relax. Take a moment to again reflect on a time you
really felt heard and supported when you shared a story with
someone.

There are several circumstances in which we can observe this.
Some may have had this experience in childhood with a caregiver,
teacher, or friend. Later, we might have this experience in more formal settings, such as a therapist's office, a religious or cultural institution, a 12-step recovery program, or other forms of group support.
There are countless others, of course. What matters is that being listened to is, in a sense, a powerful restorative practice. And as you
relax, you connect more with the person who is listening to you.

Sharing difficult and complex emotions and trauma with a
trusted person allows us to create an integrated narrative. This helps
our brains make sense of the experience by aligning our sense of
safety and understanding with the person listening to us, and then
we can move on. This is the basis for how trauma therapy works and
how many other kinds of narrative-based recovery programs work.
A trained therapist will be able to skillfully listen to your story, in an

unbiased, nonjudgmental way, and reflect back a regulated body and reaction that will help you determine a cohesive meaning.

We can't always have a trained therapist handy; however, we can offer aspects of this kind of transformational experience to each other in more everyday ways by noticing how we share, with whom, and how we feel after.

Write it!

When did sharing your story change its meaning?

Private Audience

Being read aloud to is a miniature version of what you might experience at a concert, a religious service or a sports event: the joy of an encounter magnified by the knowledge that you are sharing it with other people (in the case of reading, usually just one other person). It belongs to the valuable category of activities that combine self-embodiment and blissful self-transcendence.
—Molly Young, *New York Times* critic[23]

Silent reading only became the norm recently. For the vast majority of human history, books, texts, and stories of all kinds were read aloud and passed down through generations by rich oral traditions.

Reading aloud has many benefits. Studies at the University of South Australia show that reading aloud increases resilience,[24] and it's also been proven to increase our understanding of a story. When it comes to sharing traumatic stories, reading them aloud can provide a valuable way to embody the story, to feel what is true and how it integrates. It can result in joy.

Reading aloud can be another way of practicing sharing, something you can do with another or on your own.

Try it!

Choose a piece of your writing, or an excerpt from a passage that has meaning to you, and read it aloud. Notice how you feel in your body as the words spill out of you.

Sweep as You Go

As you find yourself listening more, your writing practice may become more supportive and more directed toward reflections and affirmations.

As you move through these pages, you may find yourself alternating between being the one sharing the story and the one listening to the story. Replenish yourself as needed.

After a meaningful conversation, pause and reflect. What do you want to carry with you? What do you want to let go of?

Write it!

What would you like to sweep away?

Flex Your Trust Muscle

By starting small and trying in a measured and
supported way, we can build our trust muscle
one rep at a time.

Many of us don't feel naturally trusting. This could be a result of
lived experience and misaligned attachment systems, the societies
we live in, or a natural part of our personality; some of us are just
more suspicious than others. What this means is that we're not all
starting at the same place when it comes to building trust.

Trusting, like listening and writing, is a practice. But, as we
explored a little earlier, practice can bring about change over time.
Trust is like a muscle: the more you use it, the stronger and more
accessible it becomes.

As Nikki Costello, internationally acclaimed Iyengar Yoga
teacher, says,

We can unpack trust by starting to create a way for people to
trust their own capacity to trust. Here are some questions we
may ask: What does trust entail? Who have you trusted?
Have you ever trusted? What is the quality of one you have
trusted? Why do you trust your dog? Why do you trust the
sea? Why do you trust the dawn? To develop trust we need to
find those things in our lives, be it another person, but maybe
not just yet. You ask what have you trusted? Can you trust
cotton? Can you trust the feel of cotton and how it will feel on
your skin? Find the things in your life you can trust, and
question how does trust come through that?

Anyone at any point can begin learning to trust. Start small. Begin by naming people, places, and things to trust. Begin with your puppy or your favorite tree, or poet, or ice cream flavor, or color. Build from there.

Write it!

Make a list of five things you trust.

Find Your Center Before You Share

An even breath can create an even mind.

Do you ever wish you had a superpower before walking into an important or intimidating conversation, stepping onto a stage, or sitting at your desk for a writing session? This sweet and simple breath is that superpower. You can practice this anywhere—while driving, on the subway platform, or at your desk. No one will know you're doing it. This is for you and you alone.

The purpose of this simple breath is to balance the mind and support a feeling of neutrality or equanimity.

Try it!

You can breathe in through your nose, out through your mouth, or in through your nose and out through your nose.

At your own rhythm, take a breath in for four counts.

Using that same rate, breathe out for four counts.

Repeat five times and then return to a natural breath.

Know Where You Begin and End

You know you are safe when you know where you are.

It's not always possible to control your external world, but you can take care of your sense of safety in the moment. This can begin by taking note of where things end and where things begin.

Find a comfortable seat and take a few rounds of breath.

Observe where you are.

Use your eyes to outline all the edges of the room. This includes any doorways and the windows, chairs, desk.

Let your gaze move slowly, like you are tracing space.

If you are outside, you can scan the horizon. Take in the natural shapes and edges of the organic objects around you. This also includes the edge of you, the outline of your body.

You can also do this with your finger and use your felt sense for where the edges are.

Write it!

Describe the edges around you—your skin, your hair, your chair, your desk. Describe in words or draw a map.

Mirror

When you take in someone else's story, it
literally becomes part of you and changes your
brain chemistry.

A recent study observing fMRI activity on a recorded brain shows
the story being told impacts listeners as much as it defines the story-
teller.[25] It's the science of empathy.

In a nutshell, here's how it works:

1. When we are listening, our brain attunes to the speaker.
2. As the speaker tells a story, our neural activity mirrors the neural
   activity of the speaker.
3. As we actively listen, our brains couple.

Another way of describing this is when we listen, our brains mirror each other. A recent study from *Trends in Cognitive Medicine*
called brain-to-brain coupling "a mechanism for creating and sharing a social world."[26] In this study researchers isolated a collection of
humans and animals in a controlled setting without distraction from
the outside world so they had uninterrupted bandwidth to listen to
each other. What these neuroscientists saw again and again was that
when areas of the speaker's brain lit up during a story, indicating an
emotional response of some kind, the listener's brain would light up
in the same place. In a nutshell, this means our brains meld.

This is why experiences like concerts, religious gatherings, and
political rallies are effective in shaping a group mindset. Stories we
take in, movies we watch, speeches we listen to, and people we listen
to impact our own brain activity. The group culture in effect functions

like a powerful editor, modifying and connecting story lines until there is one story.

This scientific phenomenon is a powerful dynamic that can work to spread stories of good—or evil. In this way, listening works as a healing agent since when we listen to a story, including our own, it can shape-shift. This is how we practice empathy, for ourselves and others.

Write it!

Describe the five people you spend most of your time with. Most likely you are already a reflection of them. How are their stories affecting you?

Trust Your Inner Editor

You don't need an agent or special masterclass; you simply need to align with an editor that is already built within.

A close friend of mine delegates all important writing decisions to her neck. That's right, not her editor, coach, or writing group but that fleshy trunk connecting her head to her shoulders receives all her most sensitive editorial questions.

After she writes a piece, she reads it back to herself, sometimes silently, sometimes aloud, paying close attention to which words or phrases elicit a vibration in her throat. She knows what to keep or delete by the vibrations she feels. If she feels a high, clear vibration, it means it's her truth (keep); if it's a low or absent vibration, it means it's not worth saying (delete/cut). This process has served her well during her accomplished writing career and has led her through some bumpy creative terrain.

Your throat is nestled in a very special place in the body. It literally connects your head to your body and acts as a member of the neck information highway. It holds up your voice like a boom operator. Despite its powerful role, it's a remarkably vulnerable, sensitive, and relatively small area. Think about all the information that needs to pass through it—between food and water going down the throat to nonstop messages to and from the brain along the spinal column to your own authentic voice rising up and down. There's a built-in editorial job there, and like any fine editor, the neck only allows the most pertinent, powerful, and truthful parts of our experience to get through. At the same time, in the nerves, muscles, and bones of our neck, we can easily feel strain coming from within us and outside of us. This reality is reflected in our language—think of colloquial phrases like *it's a pain in the neck, stick your neck out, they're neck and neck, there's a lump in my throat*, and *my heart is caught in my throat.*

Being sensitive and attuned to what our throats and necks have to say is a practice that can immensely enhance your storytelling tool kit. Here's a gentle practice to tap into the power of the throat as you seek and share your truth:

Write it!

Visualize the throat as a passageway between your mind and your body.

Describe what you see, smell, and feel as you move along the passageway. What is the environment like? Is it crowded? Empty? Fast? Slow? Is anyone else there? Use your imagination. Write freely as you explore.

Empty Out

Letting go of excess baggage creates ease and
lightness.

Every time you walk into a room or sit down, there's a whole orchestra of stories you're carrying that you might not be aware of. There might be the story you know, or you think you know, but there might be all sorts of things going on. Maybe a podcast lodges in your lungs, a conversation in your heart, an email in your lower back, and so on and so on. Since our bodies are our stories, this idea that "you are what you eat" also applies to the stories you avail yourself of (on purpose and not).

You don't need to be a writer, editor, publicist, sister, friend, parent, caretaker, therapist, or clergy member to get this. It's a human condition. We collect other people's stories. This ranges from social media chats to ancestral trauma. Most of the time, we have no idea we're carrying around other people's stories. Sometimes an obstacle to taking in others' stories is that we're full of unprocessed stories, stories that aren't even ours. It's all in there; it's all in our bodies. When we don't release stories that come in, we store them. This appears in our lives in different ways, and another way of looking at this is as symptoms of burnout, lethargy, and apathy.

A friend taught me the following practice that I use to this day, before and after I teach, or simply when I'm feeling weighed down.

Try it!

Take a seat and firmly plant your feet on the ground. Feel your seat on the earth beneath you, or whatever is comfortable for your body.

Take a few rounds of breath and notice what your breath feels like moving in your body.

Visualize something strong—like a cord, chain, crystal, or beam of light—attached to your tailbone and running all the way to the center of the earth.

Now, one by one, place every single story you are aware that you are carrying on an imaginary pulley. These could be stories you read or heard or that someone told you. These stories might have been told by people you know personally, or you could have picked these up vicariously walking through the grocery store or listening to the news. Some of these stories might even be quite old. One by one, lower them with the pulley, down to the center of the earth. Note: you're not destroying or getting rid of any of these stories; you are simply handing them over to the care of the large, all-encompassing, ever-nourishing earth.

Continue until you feel completely empty.

Now visualize a glowing orb, like a sun, about twenty feet above you. Sense its golden light. Feel its heat. Fill yourself up with this light. This is just for you; this is your energy.

Take a few breaths and come back into the room.

Write it!

What came up for you during this practice?

Use Your Antenna

You are always sensing.

What stories did you pick up today from someone you saw but didn't speak to?

Write it!

Make a list of the stories you observed.

Talk to Animals and Plants

Keeping company with nature can promote
creative flow.

Animals and plants are great sources of inspiration. They offer full-bodied attention. There is also ample research showing that spending time with animals is a wonderful way to support trauma recovery and relaxation and connection. So try it.

Hang out with an animal and write out the dialogue. What is the conversation of unconditional love?

Say hello to at least five plants and animals today, and in your journaling, practice exploring what they say back. If animals and plants aren't in your immediate vicinity, you can practice this by looking at photos, videos, or other depictions of nature.

Write it!

Write out what you heard and what you said.

Expand

Inhale and exhale to balance.

Try it!

Find a comfortable seat (or lie down or stand up, whatever is comfortable).

Take a complete inhale and exhale to balance the breath.

Then on the next inhale, sip in some air and fill up to one-third.

Retain this breath.

Take another inhale and fill up to two-thirds.

Retain this breath.

Take one more breath and fill up all the way.

Retain.

Now exhale slowly.

Repeat up to three times and then return to a natural breath.

Create a Container

I'm safe inside this container called me.
—Haruki Murakami, novelist[27]

Sometimes we get swallowed whole in conversations and lose a sense of our own space, our own story. This can happen in family dynamics, work, relationships, really anywhere where other people with needs are when we are trying to listen to them. Usually in response, we either get quiet because we're trying to help (or hide) or we shut down because we feel cornered. In all cases, it's a form of losing our voice in the moment.

This is where mindfulness can help. When we get pulled this way and that by a strong emotion, or charged detail, mindfulness can help us come back to our own breath and voice and story so we remain present with whoever we are with—and this includes ourselves.

This next practice is great for anyone who has a visual imagination. We'll use this idea of creating a container for ourselves when we're in a dense or important conversation.

Try it!

One way to prepare for emotionally charged or challenging conversations is to use your imagination to create a shield. During a draining conversation, you can imagine a colorful eggshell around you.

Use your imagination and choose the first color that comes to you and paint an egg shape in that color around your body.

Spend some time visualizing this.

Once you have the shape and color, be with it.

See what it feels like to be inside the eggshell.

See if you need to make any adjustments. For example, would you like to be in a big shell or a small shell?

Decide whether you want a hard shell or a soft shell. A hard shell may offer more protection and is a good choice when you need to focus. A softer shell is a good choice for when you know you want to communicate with others.

You will have the opportunity to adjust your shell throughout the day. For example, if someone steps into your shell, you may notice that the color is being altered. That's okay. You can simply add another coat of paint and reclaim your space.

Write it!

Describe the shell.

Where You Set Your Gaze Grows

How we use our eyes is one of the ways we
show others we are listening.

Think about what it feels like when you're talking to someone and they're looking down or away. Think about what it feels like when someone is staring or glaring or when someone is glowing or lovestruck.

Direct eye contact isn't always comfortable or possible when we're communicating with someone else. How we are holding our own gaze impacts how we take in a story. When you listen with your eyes, you literally see in terms of colors, shapes, and sizes. This can also be reflected in the quality of your gaze or where you put your attention.

Many spiritual traditions say you can see someone's soul through their eyes. We have gazed outward to ground a meditation and inward to listen to ourselves. Our gaze—how we use our eyes—is also one of the main ways we show people how we are listening. Gazing is different from looking or seeing and has little to do with the mechanical ability of the eyes. Gazing, like listening, is the quality of your attention and how you embody this with your physical posture.

Let's review some of the basic listening cues we've explored in these pages, moving from the ground up, starting at the feet to the seat to supporting a long spine, open heart, soft throat, and ultimately to eye contact. How we look at each other matters. Our eyes tell our stories and show how we are taking in stories. How do we use our eyes to listen?

Let's begin with you.

Listening with Your Eyes

Solo Practice

Grab a mirror and make eye contact with yourself for one minute. You can lock eyes with yourself or focus on one eye at a time. If this feels too intense, try focusing your gaze on your third eye or collarbone. Stay with it. Notice what you see. Try saying something nice. Try winking. Practice this for one minute.

Partner Practice

Consider inviting a friend to join you. Sit across from each other and maintain eye contact for one minute. This isn't a staring contest. Keep a gentle open gaze. It's okay to smile, or squirm. Try to stay.

Gentle reminder: if it doesn't feel authentic or comfortable to make direct eye contact, focus on the forehead, collarbone, or beyond the shoulders. It's worth noting that making eye contact doesn't have to be just about your eyes. You can make eye contact with your face, your collarbone, your shoulders. From a listening perspective, the act of facing someone and taking them in—and letting them take you in—will signal an openness, understanding, and connection. Where you direct your attention, your eyes will follow. Try this for one minute.

You may find the longer you look at someone else, the more of you is revealed.

Write it!

Notice what stories surface and what awareness emerges as you listen with your gaze. How does the way you see affect what you see? How does the quality of your gaze reveal the stories we carry?

Listen for What You Love

The greatest gift that we can give each other is the gift of our full attention without judgment.

Whether you are a mother, father, sister, brother, writer, artist, photographer, colleague, caregiver, doctor, nurse, therapist, grocery store clerk, dental hygienist, dog walker, neighbor, or even just next to someone in line at the drugstore, your presence matters. People are always sharing their stories with you, whether it's a story about their day, a story they are conveying about how they feel through their body language, or a story someone has put on the page and is sharing with you. Whether you are able to be present and listen to someone else may dramatically alter the course of someone's life. You can be the person who helps others by practicing listening; begin by practicing listening for sameness and for what you love.

Suggested guides for listening with love:

Listen for something you love or identify with.
Listen for what you want to know more about.
Do not interrupt, interject, or ask any probing, intrusive, or
    background questions.

This will help develop a habit to seek sameness and likeness, encouraging warm connection. In effect, if you act like you feel relaxed (even if you don't), your body will follow.

It is a radical act to focus on what you love. Our educational system is built on critical feedback—we are taught to seek division and to individuate. But we need to move away from a habitual fight-or-flight response toward relaxation to find harmony and derive the maximum nutrients from each other's stories.

Next time you sit down to listen to someone—this could be a live conversation or a TV show, podcast, or audiobook—take a moment to set up your body. Pay attention to the parts of the story that you identify with and what you love. Notice language that sparks a feeling or thought in you.

Notice how your body feels before, during, and after. What sensations come up?

Gut Check

Stories are just another "food" that we digest mentally and physically.

The best way to evaluate whether you're involved in a healthy and nourishing exchange is to notice how you feel twenty minutes after. You'll know how well you have digested by checking in and seeing how you feel.

Take a pause to notice how you feel in your gut. Do you feel tense? Open? Wary? Warm? Sit with your gut.

You can practice this after any conversation.

PART SIX

Grow

THE BODY BECOMES THE PEN, AND
THE WORLD BECOMES THE PAGE

I sit cross-legged on a cushion in the middle of a voluminous hall. Sunbeams stream sideways into the space from majestic floor-to-ceiling cathedral windows. My gaze tracks each body slowly filing through the double doors. I think if I look hard enough, I can capture each moment before it's gone.

It's 2016, and I'm back at the same large retreat center amid another sea of people and yoga props. But this time they're gathering in a wide circle instead of a collection of private islands. And there's another difference: I am the teacher. What remains the same is that I still feel out of my depth. Despite all my training and preparation, my habitual obsessive thinking hunkers down into a well-worn spot between my ears, running its old tapes: *What if I don't have anything to say? Who am I to think my story matters? What if I screw up? What if they're disappointed or think I'm stupid? Am I even worthy of being here?*

As I worry, people begin to find their seats, and another inner tape plays a different yet equally familiar tune, attempting to drown out the worrier with a practiced effort to plot and plan. People settle, and I map out the next two hours, visualizing, bullet point by bullet point, how I want the entire workshop to unfold. *If I hold on tightly to this plan, I can control the outcome.* For the moment my ego seems satisfied that the desired appearance of personal success will be achieved, and I direct my attention back to the people in front of me.

I take a breath and feel my seat in the present moment. I sense an energetic rustling in the room. People are creating little worlds for themselves, with blankets, bolsters, and notebooks. Some of them carry objects of meaning, such as stones, photographs, or scarves. As I relax, another voice takes the mic: *This isn't about me; they have their own stories to discover.*

I take another breath and remember a friend's encouraging words. "Remember, all of these people really want to be here," she said. "There's nothing more to do; you have already done the work. You know this stuff. Now all you need is to let go and let it unfold."

With a third round of deep breaths, I place a blanket under my cushion to add extra support and a little more comfort. I settle into the seat beneath me; it is solid and close to the ground. My eyes move across the room with intention; light is filling the space like steam. I adjust my focus to my immediate surroundings. In my little island, I have my notebook, a favorite stone, and a glass of water. I do a quick body check: *Do I have everything I need?*

I feel an inward tug, a presence from the past. My wounded, scared self alerts me to her hiding place, and I stay with her for a moment. I offer empathy and care. She has a lot to get off her chest but doesn't demand the mic; my attention is enough. With that past self now reassured, my future self is off and running, imagining that she will either be basking in bright lights and ticker tape parades or reeling from utter failure—and she is terrified of either extreme. In this present moment, I know there is another option, but the outcome is unknown: *What will happen to me if I let go of my fear? What will be left?*

A quiet hum spirals around the room as the room settles. I look around. I'm eye level with over one hundred people. I see an array of faces, some eager, some bright, some guarded, some sad—*they all want to be here.* With all those eyes looking at me, there's no escaping this moment. I can't run from my fear, so I stay. As I accept the gaze of all these people, I understand that this workshop is my offering; whatever I'm about to say and whatever the outcome, it isn't about me. My story is just one of the one hundred–plus stories that surround me, ready to find their way to light. The moment I take the focus off myself, my body relaxes. I nod silently to myself and to them, and I catch a few smiles and nods in return. I see some familiar faces, and the ones I haven't met yet already feel familiar.

I breathe and feel the breath moving through my whole body. *All of me is here.*

I rock gently backward and forward in my seat, seeking the point of balance. I close my eyes to listen before speaking, I ask for guidance. I remember the mantra my mentor shared with me beforehand: *This is service, not a performance.* As I repeat the words, I feel her with me. I'm not alone.

I let go of the script, I let go of my plans. Like an awakening volcano, the parts of my story that want to be told are pushed to the surface. I remind myself, *A story is only a gift if it wants to be shared.* I surprise myself; instead of sharing anecdotes from my professional accomplishments, I share vulnerably about my own personal story of recovery. I describe the hope I have found through sharing my story and being heard. As I breathe in, I feel my whole body present. There's no part that I'm trying to hide, fix, or force. My heart lifts, my face opens, and I'm smiling. Instead of talking to a group of strangers, I feel like I'm talking to a good friend.

It's like my body becomes the pen and the room becomes the page. I sense a new lightness and connection as my words land on each body. Words that had described shame or loneliness or unrest create bridges of understanding in ways I never could have imagined or designed. And as my body's messages become clear, there's less I need to say with my words, because the story my body is telling is supporting me too. There's a universe of dialogue happening with each nod, breath, fleeting eye contact, and gesture in the room, like a hand to someone's heart or even someone looking away.

And then I am quiet, and I offer this prompt: *What is the spark that brought you here? Why are you here?* And for the next ten minutes, we write together. I invite people to move to any part of the room they feel like, and as we move, we invite our bodies to the page first. I notice how my story changes. The spark that brings me to this present moment is not the same spark that brought me to share my story a moment ago. I meet the sea of faces around me, and we find the present moment together. In community, we begin a new page, one word at a time.

We are immersed in a deconstructed conversation, mindfully parsing the most potent morsels of experience through personal awareness practices. We notice our bodies, our breath, our comfort, our surroundings. What would it be like to bring this awareness into the world and into every encounter? What would it be like to pause and listen to myself before speaking? To check in with my body while listening with this level of care as I walk down the street, bump into neighbors, answer a text from my mother? I wonder what kind of peace might be possible.

To close our practice, I invite everyone in the room to return to their original seats. At this point, there are blankets and cushions strewn all over the place; the private islands now resemble a sleepover after a pillow fight. People find their way and reorient. Some build piles beneath them, others wrap themselves in blankets, and others are lying down. In this aggregation of people, pillows, and blankets, I prompt everyone to center their awareness around a single word that is present with them now. And then we share our words so we can compose a group poem. We are presented with a lyrical list of words: *connection, loss, gratitude, intention, inspiration, abundance, community.* I write the words on a large notepad at the front of the room. As we look back and forth between the page and each other, the energy of the group shifts; we sit with the wonder of our own insides being out in the open alongside others'. As a collective we recognize that the words themselves are not mere shapes on a page but representations of who we are, as people, in our bodies at this moment together.

Each of us, in our own quiet way, walks the path of learning and unlearning how to tolerate being seen and seeing others. As we write, we create choices of when and how to share. In this moment—with our one word on the page sitting alongside others and with our chosen visible selves befriending one another—storytelling becomes transformational healing in community. And through this cocreation, our poem shines as a beacon of wholeness that is greater than the sum of its component parts.

Off the Page and into the World

Storytelling is how we make sense of the world and forge connections with others. It makes us feel better. Storytelling, and writing, at its essence is what it means to be human. Writers often say things like, "Writing saved my life" and "Writing is like food and water." Make no mistake; this is not hyperbole. These comments are facts.

Narrative Healing is based on the premise that our stories exist to heal. They live in our bodies and have a benevolent purpose. They exist to keep us safe and support our personal well-being, our natural ecosystem, our community, and our world. We see this in nature all around us—trees shed leaves to benefit the earth, flowers release pollen to spread their seeds, and animals eliminate to fertilize the ground. Our stories exist in this same container. Not only do our stories help us individually, each story we take in and give out has the potential to help someone else—even when we don't intend it. It's automatic; each of our bodies holds a story someone else needs.

The healing power of sharing your story is not based on whether you hold a position of power in our culture, and it's not based on literary merit, nationality, race, class, religion, sexuality, gender expression, age, physical or mental ability, lifestyle, or belief system.

It goes deeper than that. It's biological. Our bodies are our stories, and we tell our stories to release them, the same way we need to sweat, eliminate, or exhale in order to be alive and to heal. How, where, and when we release them is an indication of our basic wholeness and sense of safety.

We see the benefits of sharing stories all around us—they fuel political revolutions and social justice reform. They're the glue that holds communities together, and they offer creative inspiration and joy.

When you release the story you are meant to share, it will create new meaning.

Most people I work with are coming to the page because there's something they *have* to say, something they want to shed light on, or some way they hope to help. Think back now to your intention from the first part: Has anything changed? Do you want to make any adjustments? Anything to add?

Consider taking a moment to write it down now.

———

Your stories are not designed to stay stagnant and inside. You *need* to share your stories for them to fulfill their purpose of supporting and inspiring growth. They are meant to grow, spread, connect, inspire, and thrive. This is how we grow beyond the confines of our lived experience. This is how we heal ourselves, realize our potential, and help others. We're just wired that way; we're social creatures, and we need each other to transform and ultimately find joy and bring our voices to a larger community.

This process of sharing begins within, and you're already doing it if you've gotten this far in the book. It starts with somatic awareness, compassionate listening, and building a practice and connection with a higher power. At this point, you might not even need to try; sharing could become the natural outcome of the work you have already done.

Personal writing offers limitless opportunities for personal growth and transformation, but the real magic happens when you let your story leave your body and take the risk of letting others relate to, feel, and engage with it. Melissa Febos writes, "Transforming my secrets into art has transformed me. I believe that stories like these have the power to transform the world. That is the point of literature, or at least that's what I tell my students. We are writing the history that we could not find in any other book. We are telling the stories that no one else can tell, and we are giving this proof of our survival to each other."[28]

I've seen this happen in hundreds of ways in my career working with writers at every stage of development. I've seen it in illness memoirs, manifestos, literary triumphs, and from whistleblowers, healers, and doctors. I've also seen this in groups I've led and been a part of when people share personal stories in the community, on the page, in text or email, or verbally, and *simply* in the manner they hold their bodies and share their stories silently.

Over the years I've worked with survivors of sexual assault, people living with cancer, people living with chronic pain, doctors, nurses, activists, social workers, college students, esteemed writers, homeless mothers, and many others. When they release their personal stories into the world, those narratives can act like bread crumbs for the next person on their path. I've seen this work miracles big and small; they can come in the form of a published work and in the myriad ways we communicate with each other—texts, emails, social media posts, our voices, and the way we move through the world. This is true in both low-stakes and high-stakes environments. True stories from peers sharing similar stories of survival often offer more transformative healing than any amount of expert professional advice. When a story is shared, it becomes something larger and often something unexpected.

———

While the stories and details change, what always remains the same is the stories that impact the world the most are the ones that are spoken from the heart, sharing a personal experience others can relate to. You don't need to be fancy, famous, influential, or have a lot of followers to make a global impact with your story. There is lifesaving, life-affirming, and valuable information in the stories we carry in our bodies and share with each other, whether we write a best-selling book, have a heart-centric passing conversation with a stranger, or speak our truth in a letter. Every story matters.

We are all capable of healing ourselves and each other when we harness the courage to peek out of the walls of our lived experience and be open to listening, to sharing, and to lifting each other up. When you bring your whole body along, you can dance with the world around you as it actually is.

Bringing Our Stories Out of Our Bodies and into the World

We tell our stories in order to live.
—Joan Didion[29]

For the next leg of our journey, I'm going to turn the pages over to an assortment of clients, colleagues, mentors, and collaborators. These contributions showcase inspiring examples of how sharing stories can create a sense of belonging, meaning, and community change. Each voice illustrates a meaningful example of how to pick up on cues from your body regarding what to share, when and how to share it, whether that's on the page, live in a group, or through how you move in the world. I hope they resonate with you. If they don't, please go out and listen for stories that do. There are as many paths toward sharing your healing message in the world as there are humans on the planet.

Whether we like it or not, or choose to or not, on a basic level, our stories impact the people around us. It is unavoidable. This is true of the books we read and the texts, emails, news, and any other stories that surround us. Haven't you felt the energy of someone walking in front of you? You can pick up whether they're leaving a story full of anger and resentment for you to walk over or a path of peace and joy. Similarly, when you're walking outside at night, you have an intuitive sense if someone is safe or not. When a loved one walks toward you, you can feel their energy greet you way before their arms embrace you.

Contemplate it!

Slow down right now and imagine. Can you remember a time when you saw someone you cherished across the room moving toward you and you felt it? This could be a close friend, a teacher, a partner, a furry friend—really, any being that sparks a feeling of happiness. Where did you feel it? The skin's surface? Did a smile form? Did your heart warm? This was their story meeting yours before the words came.

Write it!

Describe the experience.

Begin in Your Garden

Shelly Tygielski is the founder of Pandemic of Love,
mindfulness teacher, activist, and author of *Sit Down to Rise Up*.

We need to remember that words are purposeful, and they inspire. They don't just heal, they inspire others to move to action. They inspire others to have contemplation. They plant seeds with people. A lot of us underestimate that. Our stories, should we choose to share them, our ability to be vulnerable, is really the connecting point between the inner and the outer world.

Shelly often cites an old Buddhist proverb that says, "Tend to the area of the garden that you can reach." If we only took responsibility to tend to our gardens, our blocks, a floor in our building—forget the whole building, just one floor—or our department at work and made sure that everyone had enough, it would transform the world.

Try it!

Consider your friends, family, students, clients, neighbors, neighborhood furry friends, or barista—your immediate circle of influence. Reach out to one of them and ask them how they are doing and what would make their life easier at this moment. Listen fully to the answer. Sometimes they may not even know the answer themselves—but the answer may still arise for you. Start there. You can simply start by planting this seed. Before you know it, a forest will grow.

Reclaiming Your Story Inspires Others to Do the Same

La Sarmiento is a mindfulness, meditation, and dharma teacher.

On identities:

My immigrant parents' way of surviving was to assimilate into dominant culture in the United States. And for so long, even though I understood that I was not a white person, not a straight person, nor a cisgender person, there really was no vocabulary to describe who I was. I was being anything but myself just to feel some sense of belonging, to feel that there wasn't something innately wrong with me. I would conform to whatever society, my parents, my peers, my partners needed me to be. So, in my mid-30s, I realized that I was no longer comfortable conforming anymore. I needed to find the courage to be who I really was.

On my website, when I say that I'm an immigrant, nonbinary person of color, it's my way of putting it out there. For me, that has really been a form of liberation, truly claiming my belonging rather than depending on something external to myself to determine whether I was worthy or whether I belonged or not. We all belong. It's just inherent, our birthright.

On sharing their story in an embodied way and what that means for experience in community:

These two memories come to mind: I was a retreat manager for Tara Brach at a time when we decided to create all gender bathrooms on our retreats. I was given an opportunity to speak to the sangha as to why that was really important. For me, it was so traumatizing growing up and always being questioned about what bathroom I was in. To share my story about that experience was very vulnerable. It's often assumed that using a public restroom is not a big deal. Yet it's a big deal for folks who identify as transgender or nonbinary.

Though most of the people on the retreat were of the dominant culture, many were crying, and some even came up and hugged me afterward. I received many notes saying how much people appreciated hearing my story, how it educated them about what they often took for granted in their experience as a cisgender person. I often enter spaces wondering if there is a family or single-stalled restroom available. So, it's still a thing from when I was a little kid until now. Speaking my truth at this retreat, I felt held, supported, seen, and heard.

I was definitely shaking when I spoke up, and after experiencing the response, I felt a strong sense of *Oh, I'm a part of this sangha. There's actually a lot of love, respect, and acceptance here for me. I felt connected to the earth through a sense of groundedness and stability that has given me the courage to keep being who I am as long as I felt safe enough.*

Another example is when I managed a weeklong silent retreat with the IMCW during the week of the 2016 election. Almost everyone was shocked, disappointed, and angry in silence.

The teachers and I shared our reactions to the results. I shared that my initial response was sadness and fear, anger and disappointment. As I practiced being with it all, a voice telling me I belong no matter what arose.

I shared with the sangha that yes, with this administration there is a risk. They could annul my marriage. They could tell me what public restrooms to use. I could get killed or beaten for who I am, and you know what? I'm still going to be myself. This afternoon I am going into DC to meet with a social worker to get a letter to get top surgery. I'm going to continue living my life. I was so excited; I had wanted top surgery for so long, to align my body with how I felt inside myself. I'm just going to keep living my life, and if anyone wants to harm me in any way, whether that's through policies or physical harm or say things, because of who I am, go ahead; it's not on me. It's on them. I'm still going to lead my life and support people like myself so they can continue to be empowered and continue to be themselves. We're not going back to conforming ever again!

On the role of joy and play in their practice:

I've always loved writing dharma spoof songs. It's the best way I can teach. Who pulls out a ukulele and starts singing a spoof of Johnny Cash's "Folsom Prison Blues"? I find so many retreats so intense and so serious. Joy is the fuel to be with the suffering, with life as it is. And to not take ourselves so seriously. If you really look at human beings, it's utterly ridiculous how we view ourselves and treat each other. Writing dharma spoof songs is just a way I lighten it up. Playfulness and lightness are so important to include in our practice. What other people think of us and what we think of ourselves are just thoughts and aren't necessarily real or true.

Write it!

How do you express your identity and story? Does it empower you and others? Sharing your personal story is a form of resistance.

Sharing Your Healing Story Heals Others

Lori Meyers is a native Floridian. Her personal story about her life with MS can be found in *Voices of MS* (LaChance Publishing, 2010).

On the role of writing in her healing practice:

I really enjoy the comradery of the group, it's the validation, it's the interest and support, the feedback that I get from other writers that is the most inspiring to me. I don't really enjoy the sit at your desk and write part of it. I do that as a means to the end because I like the connection. I feel like the people I meet in writing groups are my people. They are closer to me than maybe some of the friends that I've had for many many years or some of my family even because there's a connection that is beyond the connection we have in regular life. I feel like it's a form of therapy for me, but it's better because it's not given by a therapist because the people on the other side are so similar to me. Without even knowing them. It's made me realize that. I've redefined who I want to be around and what's important to me in my experiences in the writing.

I think there's some deep-rooted pain in all of us. Somewhere in there is some pain. I think getting that pain out with a stranger / friend is remarkable. It's a stranger who becomes a friend within hours. What I've learned is that the things that are deep inside of me, things that really matter to me are not things I can really express any other way except through writing. For example, the loss of my father, I really didn't realize the depths of his impact on my life until after he died. I'm trying to sort it out, it's been eight years. It's something I can only articulate through writing because I can think about how to present it how to make it impactful when I'm writing more than when I'm talking.

I always wanted to be a writer. I always did well at it, it always came naturally to me. I release it on the page, and it's not over for me, I need to share it. That's where I get the real release. Writing it down isn't enough for me, I need to release it, I need the feedback.

I have a son who was born ten weeks early and he was in an ICU for ten weeks. The March of Dimes reached out to me at some point and asked me to be a speaker for a fundraising effort. At that point my son was 3 or 4 and doing well. I spoke for maybe five minutes at this kickoff event. I don't remember what I said. I said something like you just don't know and you just don't give up and someone came up to me after I spoke, and I was talking about my son. They had stomach cancer or something like that, and they said to me, I don't know what the connection is between what you said and what I have, but you just gave me a second chance. I'm going to give myself another chance.

I thought Wow, I did that? My pain radiated over to him, and it gave him hope. I guess that's what I'm trying to do and that's what I'm trying to do with my writing.

No matter what I do, I have to keep doing that. I have to keep sharing my pain and my relentless going back to life to trying because that's what life is. That's what everyone is doing. I have a message and I have to keep giving my message. That's what one person told me and I know there are many who have gained insight from me telling my stories.

Write about a time sharing your story helped someone else.

On the Concept of Sharing Your Story

Christina Cogswell is a deaf actor and artist living in San Francisco.

Stories are not meant to be buried in a forgotten past. Stories are meant to be shared. Giving the story a voice is very important to me. I wasn't able to voice my own stories for years due to oppression and people not believing me. When I do someone else's story, I want that person (usually the writer) to be heard and to have their story continually told.

There will always be someone who can relate to the story so they know they are not alone in their struggles, whatever it may be. It can help them feel safer to share their own story in their own time.

Being deaf is an important part of my craft because I learn, through my culture, how to read body languages and internalize it. I am able to react the way I do because of my culture. My culture and language require all of my body to communicate tone/feelings and words. My face/body is my tone, and my hands are the words.

Write it!

How do you use your whole body to communicate stories?

Share Your Voice in Community

Jamia Wilson is a writer, activist, and executive editor at Penguin Random House.

On the role of writing as a spiritual practice:

I've been brought to my knees by grief but also the pandemic and also aging and shifting ideas of what I can do. The many years I spent fueled by Red Bull and not sleeping has now led to chronic illnesses. So, I think what do I have to do differently now. The way of compassionate listening to myself didn't come easily and the simplicity of it is quite humbling. I just decided to invest in a few things. I reinvested in therapy, I hired an EMDR therapist, I got a diagnosis, that's important, where they said of course you've been unable to do things, you have complex PTSD. I hired a nutritionist and an ayurvedic coach.

I was taught that I wasn't allowed to rest. It's from my family, it's ancestral and I think it's a conditioning that comes with a Calvinist Christian conditioning. It felt like I had to apologize for resting. I have lost a sense of my core and have been living one hundred percent in my head.

I spend money and invest in myself, which is something I wouldn't do in my past—I came to consistency. What's called to my life in my forties is consistency.

I also dance.

I sometimes felt a sense of shame or disconnect that I wasn't able to connect with transcendental meditation, the kind that you sit on the mat. I felt like there was something wrong with me embodied in a nervous agitation or energy.

I was told I see in you the kind of afro indigenous barefoot in the soil that is your wisdom, and you shouldn't feel just because you're around a lot of people who have a detached way or who put a lot of value on detachment that your Sankofa energy isn't any less strong it is actually really powerful and maybe you should lean into that and that's actually my meditation right now.

There's something about the times that I have felt liberated in my soul and I'm able to see things I'm actually in movement—walking labyrinths, doing African dance, healing circles, ceremonies on water with indigenous women and baths, things like that is when I clear a lot of my stuff. The deepest things for me are more like conjurings. My grandmother used to be in a lot of what they call roots work in the south, which is in the family of voodoo, in Haiti or in the family of Santaria. They're still Christians but they're keeping those ancient ways. It's physical and it's a different kind of way. It's the spirituality of the tilling of the soil. Pick the plants and till the soil. My spirit comes to me in movement, not stillness.

I've come to realize there are certain things I do when I have writers block and things like that that come from that. For example, I have a rebounder and I jump on it when I'm blocked. I've done this since I was a kid. Now that I'm studying ayurveda and Chinese medicine I do dry brushing, oiling jumping to move that stagnation. Now I do this movement ritual which is dance and I came up with a choreography which has been really freeing and helpful. I've also been doing mobility and strength training work.

I think my place of growth and my place of real sheer truth, no ego, no bullshit, is on the page. It's something I would do if I wasn't getting paid to do it, and it's something like water and oxygen. It's something I actually need to do to self soothe, to heal, to feel catharsis. I know that if I were not to be able to write due to some limitation, I would find a way to communicate in some other way. I know it's spiritual because I know it comes from a place of seeking of truth telling truth seeking.

I do ancestral work around writing letters to departed ancestors. I've also started to do meditations when I ask a question to these ancestors and see what comes out on the page. The thing yesterday was what would you have me learn today, what would you have me do. And not to judge it or expect it to be beautiful prose, but to just let it come out. Those downloads have been really helpful. It's a feeling of knowing it comes from a place of the soul, it's contemplative, it has an awareness of evolution being essential to it. I also know it's spiritual because I don't believe I'll ever master the craft. I don't believe I'll ever reach a point of feeling I have arrived at some nexus point of writing. I always know there's a way you can stretch a little more, and not an uncomfortable stretch. There's always an edit, there's always a dive, there's always a nuance, or a tweak. This is why I like being an editor because it is a reverence to the process.

On a time that sharing her story in public was transformative:

I've been blessed to speak on many stages with people I really admire, and those moments have been really important to me, but I think the fact that I've been asked by both my mother and my grandmother to deliver their eulogies at their funerals. Those were the biggest honors of my life. To be able to have the last word and for people to entrust you to be able to tell their story in that way that has been really sacred for me.

I had a breakdown at 2:00 a.m. the night before my mother's funeral. I could not write those words. I could not form the sentences. I tried to tell my dad I couldn't do it; I wasn't going to do it. And then somehow three hours before the funeral it all came down. I printed it out, I somehow got to that church, and I delivered it. Something chemical happened there. It was powerful.

I've had lower back issues that science can explain, but there was always a sense in me that there is something about building a strong backbone. I've had some shame about it; there's something about being a woman and having a strong backbone or being Black and having a strong backbone. When I did that eulogy, there were a few men in the church who said, don't go to that pulpit, it's only for ordained preachers (i.e., men). I was going to start something. I made a discerning choice, and I made a speech about my mother as a feminist force and as a woman. I felt as I was standing there that each of my vertebrae were being put together like a Lego. Some force was putting it together. It helped me stand strong, like there was a hand on my back, I imagined it to be my mother. I could feel she was there, like the divine rod was somehow in my back. Since then, I've been really obsessed with what posture means. I've been doing ballet videos. I'm just trying to extend myself. What does it mean to knit the backbone together in a strong way. It's been really helpful to me to have this as a GPS to have a clear vision to write, to edit, to read, to express.

It was like a stake in the ground.

Write it!

Write a eulogy for someone you cherish.

Find Your Reader

Carla Zanoni is an Argentine American writer, poet, and digital media expert who was the first Latina named to the *Wall Street Journal*'s masthead; she is the first audience development strategy leader at TED.

I've often had people say to me "my audience is (insert demographic)" and then they'll say " . . . and everyone else," as if you're just going to reach the globe in that way. In a lot of ways audience development work is very scientific, it is about demographics, it is about psychographics, but at the end of the day the intuitive aspect of figuring out who your audience is asking yourself "what do I need?" What is it about what I'm writing or offering that is really answering that, and then asking who else in my life also needs that. It has to be that shared need, what is it that we have in common, and then find the way forward to meet that need. It could be a need for developing a practice, it could be a need for understanding, it could be an intellectual need to better understand how something works in the world. Get as close to the emotion as possible. The emotional space that's held in that need or want, that's the energy source. And what is the gift you are giving that person? We can't control who will respond to us because we don't even know until we put our work out into the world and share it with them until an energy exchange happens.

There is no marketing plan that you can put together that will capture that group, it's really the truth of the story that you are putting out. It's always about coming back to what is the gift that I'm giving.

What gift are you giving? Make a list of what you can offer.

On the Art of Getting Your Work into the World

Ann Tashi Slater is a writer and speaker based in Tokyo, Japan.

You are exploring your own voice and creativity by writing, and at the same time, you can put your work out into the world and connect with people who connect with what you have to say, and that feeds your writing, and you put more out into the world, and so on. You can create a nice flow. Once you start publishing, it gets easier, and you can get into a rhythm.

As writers, we work alone for the most part and sometimes feel lost. Maybe you're at your desk day after day but not getting your writing out into the world that much. What helps me is, at the beginning of every month, I think: What do I want to get done by the end of the month? Monthly goals can include the amount of writing you want to do, what you want to read, a note you want to send to a writer you admire, pieces you want to pitch or submit. And it's important not to get derailed by rejection. I like to keep in mind an image of bamboo, because bamboo bends in even the strongest wind and doesn't break. That's what we need to be like. Go with what comes and stick to your plan. If you make a plan every month, you're in control and you can keep going no matter what.

Write it!

Write your goals for the next month.

Side Lean

Find the ground to lift to the sky.

We've been doing this awhile, so let's take a stretch break. In physics, there's a principle of opposite action, or opposing forces; often we need to press down first so that we can then reach up. So the more you are connected to the ground, the higher you can reach toward the sky, toward a vastness, toward others.

It will feel effortless to release your story into the world once you find your ground.

Try it!

Stand up with your feet hip-distance apart. (You can do this seated or lying down as well.)

Inhale. Reach your arms up high, palms facing each other, like you're a superhero.

Clasp your right hand around your left wrist and side bend.

As you lean to the side, press down through your feet to lift higher.

Reach back up and release both hands.

Again, inhale and reach your arms up like you're a superhero.

Exhale. Clasp the other hand—your left hand around your right wrist—and side lean.

As you lean to the side, press down through your feet to lift higher.

Reach back up and release.

Repeat as desired.

A Story That Needs to Be Told Today

Kate Johnson is a writer, facilitator, and Buddhist meditation teacher. She leads workshops integrating meditation, restorative movement, and liberation theologies, and she works with leaders and organizations to cultivate sustainability and wise relationships in their work. She is the author of *Radical Friendship: Seven Ways to Love Yourself and Find Your People in an Unjust World*.

On motherhood and creativity:

Before my daughter was born, I missed every deadline, and after she was born, I made every one for my book. When she was three weeks old, I was getting up at 3:00 a.m. and reviewing copyedits. I would lay her on my partner's chest and then go work for a couple of hours before they both woke up.

It felt like . . . not urgency in the white supremacy form of the word, but urgency in the sense that time is so precious and when there's someone so small in my life, I'm so acutely aware of the passage of time and of how much actually changes in a year. The changes that happen between ages thirty-seven and thirty-eight aren't a big deal to us, but four weeks to fourteen weeks is phenomenal. It gave me the fire of "the time is now."

What I'm learning too about my own storytelling and my own writing process is that there's a story that needs to be told today. If I don't write it or record it, or tell it in some way, it's gone. If I sit down two weeks later to try to write that story it may or may not still be. So that's been part of my process too, that everything's not going to get written down.

On listening to ancestors:

I've been revising and writing what it means to be a mother in my family lineage. A little bit into my pregnancy I had an evening that I can only describe as a generational download. I was lying on my bed relaxing, and I could suddenly see a series of doors opening up behind me. The feeling was of being connected into something that went further back. Like a long story and pushing that story ahead in that particular way.

I'm learning more and more through parenting my kiddo how I myself was parented. Realizing that the stories I was told about what a mother is and what she does isn't necessarily the kind of mother I want to be, nor the kind of mother I want to model for my child. A lot of it has to do with martyrdom and self-sacrifice and the giving up of dreams. What I learned as a kid is that the work of a mother is to abandon herself. Not only am I learning slowly and with great determination that that's not necessarily true. I really feel motivated to show my child that our well-being is not a zero-sum game. When I thrive, she thrives and vice versa. It also means not using my child as an excuse to not continue to live my life. It's scary to continue to grow, it's scary to put new work into the world and start new projects. It would be easy to blame it on these relationships, in terms of I can't continue to grow and change because I need to focus on this small being. I don't believe that story anymore.

I know that many of my ancestors had dreams that they weren't able to realize for a variety of reasons. A lot of them had to do with the societal injustices that are still present but were even more violent and debilitating when they lived. Like

I learned that my uncle Jimmie who was a doorman in New York who moved from Honduras always had a book at his desk when he was working. He used to love to go to the theater. He was a man who loved letters and performance. I think about my Grandma Kathleen who was a domestic worker and also an activist. She took off on a whim to the March on Washington. And was a fierce advocate for her kids and their education to the point of using her employer's address so she could send her kids to school in a nicer neighborhood.

So, part of what feels like rewriting, is just doing it for the team. When putting my voice out and being heard feels really scary when there's fear of criticism or not being good enough or smart enough . . . the thought this is not just about me is incredibly liberating.

Write it!

Write the story that needs to be told today.

Writing to Heal

Meghan Zipin is the author of *First Light* (April 2023), a poetry collection chronicling her survival of the Boston Marathon bombing and journey into motherhood.

For me writing comes and goes. I never formally think of it as a healing process. In certain moments it simply feels like I need to say something, or I might explode. That need usually finds its way to my phone and those notes ultimately turn into essays, poem prompts or poetry. Lots of my writing happens in the middle of the night when I can't sleep or in the moments where my kiddos are occupied. If I see something during the day that I want to write about later, I keep a running list of interesting things, that way I never feel the pressure of coming up with a topic. I also find that writing as I'm called eliminates the pressure of "needing to write."

Initially, writing didn't come with an intent to share. It just came as a place I could be anonymous; I didn't have to endure the person receiving the information, which sometimes was the looks on their face, the startlement, the questions. It filled time that otherwise was really hairy for me, like the middle of the night. And in comparison to a therapeutic relationship, there was no ask that I walked away with, like *and now* . . . I could just leave it and walk away.

It took me a long time in therapy to talk about anything more than the weather, but every time I left, my therapist at the time would give me a Post-it Note. With hindsight, it was meant to be a guide, like something solid to hold on to. It was also something meant to help me personally to take the next step toward whatever that inch stone was. With writing, nobody gave me a Post-it Note after. It's just "I'm closing this document because I personally feel done with this."

I felt like my fingers could keep up closer to the pace of my thoughts than my verbal communication. My verbal communication was so stymied in a traumatic freeze that I could not say anything, but my brain was going a million miles per hour.

It's hard for me to separate writing from trauma recovery because it has been such an integral part of my recovery process. Anytime I write anything now, I still revel in the anonymity of it. I look to write things that either I would have wanted to hear, or I couldn't say, or I wish someone had said to me. It all kind of rests in that place for me.

My writing voice is my most authentic. I am in control of releasing it without the demands of anybody else. Part of verbalizing in many ways is reciprocal and there's a pressure that comes with that. It's probably why I love spoken word poetry. I want someone to go up there and say their most inner authentic self and perform in a way they would want to say it but probably couldn't in a normal conversation. I love listening to the performance and watching someone just walk away. No Post-its. You just get to do it and go.

Write it!

Why do you write?

When You Shine a Light on Others, You Shine Too

Be a citizen among citizens.

Sometimes the best place to begin is by offering service to others. Service can be a good starting point if you are feeling anxious, alone, afraid, blocked, or bored, or if you're feeling scattered, joyful, or overstimulated by excitement and abundance. When all else fails, supporting another person can be a good first step.

In literary communities, this concept has been called *literary citizenship*. This essentially means engaging in any activity relating to or supporting the writing life, aside from the act of writing. There are many activities to choose from, including buying a book at your local bookstore, borrowing a book from your local library, writing a review and sharing recommendations with your networks, and attending a book event or signing.

These efforts are most impactful for you and others when you begin from an authentic place. My favorite practice to inspire literary citizenship comes from my friend and literary impresario Jennifer Baker. Jenn is an author, editor, activist, and advocate for all things relating to storytelling. She's also the creator of the visionary podcast *Minorities in Publishing*. Her enthusiasm is contagious, and I'd like to turn this next prompt over to her and share her words.

Try it!

As Jenn says, "I like to think, 'What is the best compliment that someone can give to you?' Write it down. Think of the kind of thing that someone can say that can change everything for you. Now share that compliment with someone else."

Share that compliment with your chosen person. You can do this in the silent sanctity of your own thoughts or you can write to them, speak to them, or say it with your smile. You choose.

The End Is Also a Beginning

Nikki Costello is an educator with thirty years of teaching and training experience in the yoga and wellness industry.

On service:

When I was living in the ashram, which is of course a spiritual community, the focus of the ashram was service. A path of service can be what opens up the messy, the history, the understanding of story because you're in action serving others or serving a mission.

Some people start knowing they want to have an embodied practice or some kind of engagement, but for others it can begin with doing this thing [service], like waking up every morning and cooking breakfast and through that the unraveling or the revealing takes place.

Some people don't know how to begin with themselves, but know they want to get on in there and get their hands dirty and be engaged with others and then through that know themselves.

How do we know we're making the right decision when so many decisions are made because of fear or avoiding pain or avoiding suffering or attempting not to repeat a pattern or behavior or addiction. If we're in charge of navigating our own healing life, what in fact supports that? In my experience service, just getting in there and doing for others helps me realize that the giving aspect, the outpouring of my own love and attention is healing.

There Is No Destination

We learn that there is no peace walk; that peace is the walk;
that there is no happiness walk; that happiness is the walk.
We walk for ourselves. We walk for everyone always
hand in hand. Walk and touch peace every moment.
Walk and touch happiness every moment.
Each step brings a fresh breeze. Each step makes a flower
bloom under our feet. Kiss the Earth with your feet.
Print on Earth your love and happiness. Earth will be
safe when we feel in us enough safety.
—Thich Nhat Hanh[30]

How you walk is how you write, how you write is how you think, how you think is how you talk to yourself, how you talk to yourself is how you talk to others, how you listen to yourself is how you listen to others, and so on. In other words, and it bears repeating, *How you do anything is how you do everything.* A walking meditation is a wonderful way to practice mindfulness in almost any moment and can provide a guide to how to walk away from this book and then return as you are inspired.

It also provides an alternative to meditation for when the mind or the body cannot sit still with closed eyes for any reason. You can try this on the sidewalk, at the subway station, in the woods, in your workplace, in your home, during a gathering—really anywhere out in the world moving around.

Try it!

Choose a location. Ideally, find a place where you have ten to thirty feet in front of you to move through.

Feel the ground beneath you.

Set a soft gaze in front of you.

Take a step forward and sense the periphery, and you will keep your gaze in front of you.

Pause.

Take another step.

Continue.

With each step, observe and come back to the present moment. If you like, you can repeat the mantra *I am here* with each step, or anything else that calls to you.

There is no destination. There is no hurry. Walking is not the means; it is an end to itself. This is just like writing when we are writing mindfully. Writing itself is the destination. It is the practice. With this walking meditation, we can feel how this is possible.

Continue in this manner until you get to the end of your path. Then turn around and come back. This can also be done moving in a circle, just like this book.

Modification for sitting or lying down

Using two fingers, take one step and then another, *walking* your fingers along a surface in front of you. You can also use your eyes or your imagination to visualize moving in the world.

Write it!

Make a list of ways of sharing your story (that isn't writing a book).

I'll begin. Here are a few more ways to share your story:

Create a newsletter.

Write a blog.

Write a letter and send it.

March in a protest.

Write a letter and don't send it.

Walk in your truth.

Post on social media.

Walk into a room with awareness.

Be present when you answer the phone.

Pause before you reply to a text or email.

Listen to your body.

Your turn. Write three more.

The Message That's Needed Most

I have a friend who likes to say, "Help is always available as long as you don't demand where it comes from." Our stories work this way too. We can't always know which ones will be the ones that spark our own healing or help another, but as long as they are shared wholeheartedly, they will land on the right body and release the message that's needed most. It's often a message that far exceeds what we think we are asking for.

For our final moments, I'll turn the pages to you.

Try it!

Find a comfortable seat.

Take a break from the screen, from the page, this book, and all effort.

Go inward.

Go ahead and consider closing your eyes.

Pause.

Bring one hand to your heart and the other hand to your belly.

Take a few deep breaths.

Consider devoting the benefits of this journey to someone you know who needs this message. That person could be you.

Write it!

You have the last word.

Imagine yourself many months from now, a full season away, when you might need this message. Imagine what that day might look like. Perhaps it's a packed workday, or you find yourself juggling many needs; perhaps you're not feeling well, or perhaps you're cele-brating a personal triumph. Bring a clear image of yourself.

What do you want to remember from this experience?

What do you want your future self to know? Write it down now.

When you're ready, send it out into the universe in a way that feels authentic to you. You might write a letter, fold it into an enve-lope, and mail it; you could record it; or you could place it in a time capsule. You might bury it or burn it or wrap it up and tie it in a bow. The options are limitless, and they are yours.

Gratitude and Next Steps

Dear Reader,

Thank you for sharing your precious time, attention, and energy with me. You inspire me, and it's an honor to be on this path with you.

If you're interested in diving in deeper, I'm sharing a selection of books that have resonated with me during my journey creating this book. I hope they are helpful to you and will be companions to you on your creative and healing journey. If my personal library doesn't support your needs, or if I have left out resources that are important to you, I hope you will seek out what will best serve you.

This offering is a path, not a checklist, and it's meant to be done with others. I hope you'll join me and the Narrative Healing Community (www.narrativehealing.com) as we continue to unlock the healing power of storytelling in our changing world. My intention is to cocreate space to share resources, experiences, challenges, and joys in community with one another.

With great love and appreciation,

Lisa

Resources

I am not a trained professional or licensed therapist. If you or someone you know is in need of immediate assistance, please call any one of these professional hotlines.

Call 911 and see urgent care. You can also try these hotlines: 1-888-NYC-WELL or the new 988 number instead of 911 crisis text line.

National Suicide Prevention Hotline, 24-7: 800-273-8355; 888-628-9454 (en español)

Department of Mental Health Access and Crisis Line, 24-7: 800-854-7771

Substance Abuse Mental Health Services Administration, 24-7: 800-662-4357

Further Reading

This is a selection of books that have sustained and inspired me while writing this book. I hope they will enrich your creative path and lead you on to explore more resources.

TRAUMA HEALING

Dana, Deb. *Anchored: How to Befriend Your Nervous System Using Polyvagal Theory.* Sounds True, 2021.

Herman, Judith. *Trauma and Recovery: The Aftermath of Violence—from Domestic Abuse to Political Terror.* Basic Books, 1997.

Khoudari, Laura. *Lifting Heavy Things: Healing Trauma One Rep at a Time.* Lifetree Media, 2021.

Levine, Peter A. *Healing Trauma: Restoring the Wisdom of the Body.* Sounds True, 2008.

Levine, Peter A. *Waking the Tiger: Healing Trauma.* North Atlantic Books, 1997.

Menakem, Resmaa. *My Grandmother's Hands: Racialized Trauma and the Pathway to Mending Our Hearts and Bodies.* Central Recovery, 2021.

Van Der Kolk, Bessel A. *The Body Keeps the Score: Brain, Mind, and Body in the Healing of Trauma.* Penguin, 2015.

WRITING AND HEALING

Aronie, Nancy. *Memoir as Medicine: The Healing Power of Writing Your Messy, Imperfect, Unruly (but Gorgeously Yours) Life Story.* New World Library, 2022.

Charon, Rita. *Narrative Medicine: Honoring the Stories of Illness.* Oxford University Press, 2008.

DeSilver, Albert. *Writing as a Path of Awakening: A Year to Becoming an Excellent Writer and Living an Awakened Life.* Guilford, 2016.

Hannan, Judith. *The Write Prescription: Telling Your Story to Live with and Beyond Illness.* Archer, 2015.

Jamison, Leslie. *The Empathy Exams: Essays.* Graywolf, 2014.

Mehl-Madrona, Lewis. *Narrative Medicine: The Use of History and Story in the Healing Process.* Bear, 2007.

Ofri, Danielle. *What Doctors Feel: How Emotions Affect the Practice of Medicine.* Beacon, 2014.

Pennebaker, James. *Expressive Writing: Words That Heal.* Idyll Arbor, 2014.

Remen, Rachel Naomi. *Kitchen Table Wisdom: Stories That Heal.* Riverhead Books, 1996.

MEMOIRS

Angelou, Maya. *I Know Why the Caged Bird Sings.* Random House, 2009.

Bailey, Elisabeth Tova. *The Sound of a Wild Snail Eating.* Algonquin Books, 2016.

Bauby, Jean-Dominique. *The Diving Bell and the Butterfly: A Memoir of Life in Death.* Vintage, 1998.

Burke, Tarana. *Unbound: My Story of Liberation and the Birth of the Me Too Movement.* Flatiron Books, 2021.

Carroll, Rebecca. *Surviving the White Gaze: A Memoir.* Simon & Schuster, 2021.

Didion, Joan. *The Year of Magical Thinking*. Knopf Doubleday, 2007.

Ford, Ashley C. *Somebody's Daughter: A Memoir*. Flatiron Books, 2022.

Gay, Roxanne. *Hunger: A Memoir of (My) Body*. Harper Perennial, 2018.

Jamison, Kay Redfield. *An Unquiet Mind: A Memoir of Moods and Madness*. Vintage, 1996.

Jaouad, Suleika. *Between Two Kingdoms: A Memoir of a Life Interrupted*. Random House, 2022.

Karr, Mary. *The Liar's Club: A Memoir*. Penguin, 2005.

Khapour, Porochista. *Sick: A Memoir*. Harper Perennial, 2018.

Mandel, Sarah. *Little Earthquakes: A Memoir*. Harper, 2023.

Newton, Maud. *Ancestor Trouble: A Reckoning and a Reconciliation*. Random House, 2022.

Rapp, Emily. *The Still Point of the Turning World*. Penguin, 2014.

Salzberg, Sharon. *Faith: Trusting Your Own Deepest Experience*. Riverhead Books, 2003.

Shapiro, Dani. *Devotion: A Memoir*. Harper Perennial, 2011.

Shapiro, Dani. *Inheritance: A Memoir of Genealogy, Paternity, and Love*. Knopf Doubleday, 2020.

Silver, Elizabeth. *The Tincture of Time: A Memoir of (Medical) Uncertainty*. Penguin, 2018.

Solnit, Rebecca. *Recollections of My Nonexistence: A Memoir*. Penguin, 2021.

Walls, Jeanette. *The Glass Castle: A Memoir*. Scribner, 2006.

PERSONAL ESSAY COLLECTIONS

DiAngelo, Robin. *White Fragility: Why It's So Hard for White People to Talk about Racism*. Beacon, 2020.

Febos, Melissa. *Body Work: The Radical Power of Personal Narrative*. Catapult, 2022.

Febos, Melissa. *Girlhood*. Bloomsbury, 2022.

Koven, Suzanne. *Letter to a Young Female Physician: Notes from a Medical Life*. W. W. Norton, 2022.

Oliver, Mary. *Upstream: Selected Essays*. Penguin, 2019.

Solnit, Rebecca. *The Faraway Nearby*. Penguin, 2014.

Solnit, Rebecca. *A Paradise Built in Hell: The Extraordinary Communities That Arise in Disaster*. Penguin, 2010.

Strayed, Cheryl. *Tiny Beautiful Things: Advice from Dear Sugar Anniversary Edition*. Knopf Doubleday, 2022.

Wang, Esme Weijun. *The Collected Schizophrenias: Essays*. Graywolf, 2019.

POETRY I TURN TO

Angelou, Maya. *Poems*. Bantam, 1997.

Clifton, Lucille. *Blessing the Boats: New and Selected Poems 1988–2000*. BOA Editions.

Diaz, Natalie. *When My Brother Was an Aztec*. Copper Canyon, 2012.

Harjo, Joy. *Conflict Resolutions for Holy Beings: Poems*. W. W. Norton, 2017.

Howe, Marie. *Magdalene: Poems*. W. W. Norton, 2017.

Knott, Bill. *I Am Flying into Myself: Selected Poems, 1960–2014*. Farrar, Straus and Giroux, 2018.

Myles, Eileen. *Evolution*. Grove, 2018.

Oliver, Mary. *Felicity: Poems*. Penguin, 2015.

Parker, Morgan. *There Are More Beautiful Things Than Beyoncé*. Tin House, 2017.

Rankine, Camille. *Incorrect Merciful Impulses*. Copper Canyon, 2016.

Spaulding, Holly Wren. *If August*. Alice Greene, 2017.

Vuong, Ocean. *Night Sky with Exit Wounds*. Copper Canyon, 2016.

Zipin, Meghan. *First Light*. Nymeria, 2023.

ON CREATIVITY AND CRAFT

Cameron, Julia. *The Artist's Way*. Tarcher Perigree, 2016.

Dillard, Annie. *The Writing Life*. Harper Perennial, 2013.

Gilbert, Elizabeth. *Big Magic: Creative Living Beyond Fear*. Bloomsbury, 2016.

Goldberg, Natalie. *Writing Down the Bones*. Shambhala, 2016.

Gornick, Vivian. *The Situation and the Story: The Art of Personal Narrative*. Farrar, Strauss and Giroux, 2001.

King, Stephen. *On Writing: A Memoir of the Craft*. Scribner Reissue, 2002.

Shapiro, Dani. *Still Writing: The Perils and Pleasures of a Creative Life*. Grove, 2014.

MINDFULNESS, YOGA, AND MEDITATION

Benson, Herbert. *The Relaxation Response*. William Morrow Paperbacks, 2000.

Brach, Tara. *Radical Acceptance*. Random House, 2004.

Cardoza, Nicole. *Mindful Moves: Kid-Friendly Yoga and Peaceful Activities for a Happy, Healthy You*. Storey, 2021.

Chodron, Pema. *The Wisdom of No Escape: And the Path of Loving Kindness*. Shambhala, 2018.

Connelly, Dianne M. *All Sickness Is Homesickness*. Wisdom Well, 2014.

Cope, Stephen. *Yoga and the Quest for True Self*. Bantam, 2000.

Ellison, Koshin Paley. *Wholehearted: Slow Down, Help Out, Wake Up*. Wisdom, 2019.

Hanh, Thich Nhat. *You Are Here: Discovering the Magic of the Present Moment*. Shambhala, 2010.

Hanh, Thich Nhat. *Your True Home: The Everyday Wisdom of Thich Nhat Hanh*. Shambhala, 2011.

Hirsey, Tricia. *Rest Is Resistance: A Manifesto*. Little, Brown, 2022.

Johnson, Kate. *Radical Friendship: Seven Ways to Love Yourself and Find Your People in an Unjust World*. Shambhala, 2021.

Kane, Yoon Im. *The Mindfulness Workbook for Depression*. Rockridge Press, 2020.

McCreary, Crystal. *Little Yogi Deck: Simple Yoga Practices to Help Kids Move through Big Emotions.* Bala Kids, 2021.

Nichtern, Ethan. *The Road Home: A Contemporary Exploration of the Buddhist Path.* Northpoint, 2016.

Owens, Lama Rod. *Love and Rage: The Path of Liberation through Anger.* North Atlantic Books, 2020.

Palmer, Parker. *Let Your Life Speak: Listening for the Voice of Vocation.* Jossey-Bass, 1999.

Parker, Gail. *Restorative Yoga for Ethnic and Race-Based Stress and Trauma.* Singing Dragon, 2021.

Pransky, Jillian. *Deep Listening: A Healing Practice to Calm Your Body, Clear Your Mind, and Open Your Heart.* Rodale, 2017.

Salzberg, Sharon, *Lovingkindness: The Revolutionary Art of Happiness.* Shambhala Classics, 1995.

Scurlock-Durana, Suzanne. *Reclaiming Your Body: Healing from Trauma and Awakening Your Body's Wisdom.* New World Library, 2017.

Stanley, Tracee. *Radiant Rest: Yoga Nidra for Deep Relaxation and Awakened Clarity.* Shambhala, 2021.

Tippett, Krista. *Becoming Wise: An Inquiry into the Mystery and Art of Living.* Penguin, 2017.

Tygielski, Shelly. *Sit Down to Rise Up: How Radical Self-Care Can Change the World.* New World Library, 2021.

Williams, Justin Michael. *Stay Woke: A Meditation Guide for the Rest of Us.* Sounds True, 2020.

Acknowledgments

I'm grateful, first and foremost, for the part of me and of you that is indestructible, whole, intact and possesses a bottomless well of resilience. This part is always there, always reliable and true, and it fuels me.

I have had the best time making this book, and I am deeply thankful for the scores of people who made this journey possible. I'm especially grateful to my outstanding agent, Gareth Esersky, who believed in this project from the start, opened doors I never even dared knock on, and is a joy to work with, and to my brilliant, kind, and openhearted editor, Renee Sedliar, who has been a true partner and offered tremendous care and guidance. Working with the incomparable team at Hachette Go has been a dream come true. Many thanks to publisher Mary Ann Naples and everyone in editorial, including Alison Dalafave and Cisca Schreefel. Thank you to Amanda Kain for the beautiful cover, and thank you to the publicity and marketing team of Michelle Aielli, Michael Barrs, Kindall Gant, and Ashley Kiedrowski; huge thanks to Tiffany Rotach and Jen Patten who produced and directed the audiobook. The care and thoughtfulness brought to each step of publication blew me away.

Creating Narrative Healing and teaching this program has sustained and inspired me in profound ways. Thank you to Kripalu Center for Yoga & Health, Omega Institute for Holistic Studies, and Wesleyan University for taking a chance on me and supporting this work from the very beginning. I'm beyond grateful to the Narrative Healing community for providing me with a purpose and home; thank you to everyone who shows up and makes this work possible. This community is a cocreation, and I owe everything to you.

Thank you to the many stewards who shepherded this project, including Lexy Bloom, who has been a champion of this book before a single word was written. I never would have gotten to this point without a small cluster of trusted readers who poured love all over early drafts and gave me the courage to keep going, especially Mara Dowdall, Elizabeth Keenan, Ann Tashi Slater, and Emma Weinert. Many thanks to Laura Khoudari, Jennifer Kurdyla, Eva Ludwig, Makeba Rasin, Benish Shah, and Julia Sedlock for offering essential feedback and guidance at critical stages.

Thank you to my teachers, who encouraged me and helped me discover my voice, especially Nikki Costello, Anne Greene, Julie Mellk, Bob Montera, and the late Victor Navasky. Thank you to my mentors Brette Popper, Jillian Pransky, and Ellen Scordato, who believed in me until I believed in myself; their grace, confidence, and love helped me more than I can describe.

Heartfelt thanks to everyone who appears in this book. I thank you for sharing your experiences and lending your voice to these pages. This book would not be possible without your wisdom (see complete bios at end of the book).

I also want to thank the special support and guidance I received from 192 Books (especially Evan Dent), Cali Alpert, Tina Andreadis, Charles Barber, Molly Barton, Catherine Birndorf, Rachel Bloom, Jessie Braun, Sadie Brightman, Emily Brimmer, Chris Cavanagh, Blair Cobb, Ali Cramer, Lee Delegard, Thomas Droge, Moira Cleary-Dwyer, Joyce Englander Levy, Laura Evensen, Sherman Ewing, Melissa Febos, Alison Fox, Courtney Greenhalgh, Lucia Green-Weiskel, Courtney Greenhalgh Judith Hannan, Abby Hirsch, Perry Pigeon Hooks, Suleika Jaouad, Jenny Jackson, Millie Jackson, Neta Katz, Kate Lee, The Li.st, Katharine Lord Sarah

Mandel, Susan McPherson, Suzi Nauser, Ethan Nichtern, Erin O'Flynn, Kelly Prentice, Andrew Rivera, Sally Roberts, Heang Rubin, Nikki Rubin, Danielle Samalin, Dani Shapiro, Holly Wren Spaulding, Sylvia Sutton, Kim Thai, Shelly Tygielski, Emilie Unterweger, Jamia Wilson, Justin Michael Williams, Carla Zanoni, and Meghan Zipin.

With all my heart, I thank everyone on my gratitude list, CM, SHAS, and WBBW, and countless others. I owe my life to your kindness, generosity, care, and power of example. I'm grateful to all my ancestors, real and chosen, who offered inspiration, warning, guidance, and protection. I'm especially grateful to my great-grandmother Beatrice, my grandma Thelma, my aunt Roselle, my beloved Fifi, and my spirit animal Stella Loretta.

Thank you to my family of origin. My fabulous mother, Sylvia Ann Hewlett, who shows me by example how to lead a creative life, and when I asked, "Am I setting the bar too high?" replied without missing a beat, "Where else are you going to set it? Don't you dare set it low!" My father, Richard Weinert, who has always been my loudest cheerleader; read to me every night while I was growing up and once spent six and a half hours helping me pick out the perfect stuffed animal. My outrageously wonderful siblings, Shira, David, Adam, and Emma, my best friends, life partners, and forever allies. Huge thanks to new members of my family through marriage and births; Alex, Amalia, Anais, Anika, August, Luana, and R.B.; and Bennett, Colin, Jen Millie, and Sylvia for your love and support.

I'm thankful for the throbbing, irrepressible heart that is New York City, my home. I just can't quit you. This city brings me to my knees, lifts my heart, and offers me endless opportunities to grow, practice flexibility, and confront and take in humanity.

Last, but not least, I am deeply grateful to my husband, Barry Sutton, and our little family, who have brought untold joy and unconditional love into my life and have given me a nourishing ground to launch from, return to, rest on, and belong to.

Contributor Bios

Delia Ahouandjinou is a manual therapist. She proposes visceral manipulation, is certified in craniosacral therapy, and has adapted her practice to distance healing. Her career arose from her experience as a dancer and her personal healing journey. Nourished by an ongoing multidimensional and multicultural research of healing modalities, Delia facilitates mind-body harmony and deep transformational healing.

Website: manualtherapynyc.com

Jennifer Baker was named the 2019 Publishers Weekly Star Watch "SuperStar" because her "varied work championing diversity in publishing has made her an indispensable fixture in the book business." Jennifer is the editor of *Everyday People: The Color of Life—A Short Story Anthology* with Atria Books (an imprint of Simon & Schuster). Her YA novel *Forgive Me Not* is published by Nancy Paulsen Books (an imprint of Penguin Random House) in August 2023.

Jennifer is a publishing professional with more than twenty years' experience in a range of roles (editorial, production, media) and is an instructor for Bay Path University's Creative Nonfiction MFA, as well as the creator and host of the podcast *Minorities in Publishing* (a finalist for the Digital Book World Best Use of Podcasting in Book Marketing in 2018, 2019, and 2020).

Website: www.jennifernbaker.com
Instagram: @jbakernyc

Sadie Brightman is the award-winning founder and executive director of Middlebury Community Music Center, a nonprofit music school in Vermont; she is also an applied music faculty member at Middlebury College. Her work as a musician, community leader, and educator is grounded in deep reflection, including close examinations of the systemic and historical constraints on creativity, especially for those in marginalized social groups. Sadie's interest in the intersection of performance psychology, creativity, empowerment, identity, and gender informs her writing, teaching, program development, and community-building work.

As a classical pianist, Sadie has performed as a soloist and collaborator in concerts throughout New England and abroad, and as a keyboard player and vocalist with many artists and groups, from Anaïs Mitchell to Guster. A deep believer in the power of music to move, Sadie contributed piano score work to the Oscar-nominated film *The Lost Daughter.*

Sadie has a master of music degree in piano performance from the Longy School of Music of Bard College and a BA in music from Wesleyan University. With more than two decades of piano-teaching experience, Sadie currently works closely with the Golandsky Institute, studying and teaching the work of Dorothy Taubman, a pianist and teacher instrumental in incorporating the physiological basis for movements that optimize technique and artistry at the piano. In all her endeavors, Sadie is passionate about promoting health, joy, and well-being in the arts.

Websites: www.sadiebrightman.com
Instagram: @sadiebrightman

Dan Cayer is a writer and teacher committed to helping others find freedom from pain and create a sane relationship with their bodies.

After a serious injury left him unable to work or take care of himself, he began studying the Alexander Technique. He is also a longtime Buddhist meditator and teacher. Dan frequently writes about the intersection of health and spirituality. He is at work on a book about how to transform the experience of pain and illness into a path of openness and kindness. He lives in the Hudson Valley with his wife and two daughters.

Newsletter: dancayer.substack.com

Website: www.dancayer.co

Christina Marie Cogswell is an actor, stage manager, and collaborative writer. She has worked with New York Deaf Theater, Public Works, Rochester Institute for Technology, National Technical Institute for the Deaf, and the National Theatre of the Deaf. She also has experience working in theater and television and is a dog walker in San Francisco, California.

Stephen Cope is a best-selling author and scholar who specializes in the relationship between the Eastern contemplative traditions and Western depth psychology. Among his seminal works in this area are *Yoga and the Quest for the True Self*, *The Wisdom of Yoga*, and *The Great Work of Your Life*. His most recent work, *Deep Human Connection*, is an examination of the psychology, neurobiology, and spirituality of deep human connection and the imperatives of human attachment—an issue of great importance to both the Eastern and Western traditions.

For almost thirty years, Stephen has been scholar-in-residence at the renowned Kripalu Center for Yoga and Health, the largest center for the study and practice of yoga in the Western world. Kripalu hosts almost fifty thousand guests a year in its many yoga, meditation, and personal growth programs. It is located on a sprawling two-hundred-acre estate in Stockbridge, Massachusetts. In addition to his role as scholar-in-residence, Stephen is the founder and former director of the Kripalu Institute for Extraordinary Living. It is one of the world's most influential research institutes examining the effects and mechanisms of yoga and meditation and hosts a team of researchers from Harvard Medical School, University of Connecticut, University of Pennsylvania, and many more.

Stephen is the recipient of both a Telly and an Apple award for his work. In its twenty-fifth anniversary edition, *Yoga* named him one of the most influential thinkers, writers, and teachers on the current American yoga scene.

Website: www.stephencope.com

Instagram: @stephen_cope_author

Nikki Costello is an educator with thirty years of teaching and training experience in the yoga and wellness industry. She works at the intersection of social justice and yoga, with a focus on facilitating new models of embodied leadership. Nikki is a senior Iyengar yoga teacher (level 3 CIYT) and a certified yoga therapist (C-IAYT). In 2013–2014, she was a contributing editor at *Yoga Journal*, writing the magazine's "Basics Column," and in 2016, Nikki was named one of the 100 Most Influential Teachers in America. She is the featured Iyengar yoga teacher on GLO. Nikki holds an MA in traditions of yoga and meditation from SOAS, University of London, and is a PhD candidate at the California Institute of Integral Studies. Since 2020, she has taught weekly online yoga and meditation classes at Nikki Costello | The Practice.

Website: www.nikkicostello.com

Instagram: @nikki_costello

Jessica Kung Dreyfus is an internationally renowned educator, artist, author, and speaker. She has trained and inspired thousands of people to deepen their connection to their purpose. She has dedicated twenty years to the study of art, architecture, meditation, yoga philosophy, asana, and Sanskrit. As part of her intensive training in meditation, Jessica completed a year-and-a-half-long silent retreat with her husband. She holds a BA cum laude in architecture from Yale University and an MFA from California College of the Arts.

Websites: www.makeconscious.com

Instagram: @makeconscious

Rabbi David A. Ingber serves as the senior director of Jewish life at the 92Y and is the founding rabbi of Romemu, the largest Renewal synagogue in the United States. Rabbi Ingber founded Romemu in NYC in 2006, following his ordination by Rabbi Zalman Schachter-Shalomi, founder of the Jewish Renewal movement. Over the past decade, Romemu has grown into a weekly home for thousands of people, with a membership of more than one thousand in its two physical locations (Manhattan and Brooklyn) and a growing online global membership. Rabbi Ingber also founded Romemu Yeshiva, the first fully egalitarian yeshiva (immersive learning center) dedicated to mystical and meditative Jewish learning and practice.

Website: www.romemu.org/rabbi-david-ingber

Kate Johnson works at the intersections of spirituality, social action, embodiment, and creativity. She has been practicing Buddhist meditation in the Western Insight/Theravada tradition since her early twenties and was empowered as an independent dharma teacher through Spirit Rock Meditation Center's four-year retreat teacher training in 2020. She holds a BFA in dance from the Alvin Ailey School and Fordham University and an MA in performance studies from New York University. As a meditation teacher, Kate leads programs integrating meditation, restorative movement, and liberation theologies. She is the author of *Radical Friendship: Seven Ways to Love Yourself and Find Your People in an Unjust World*.

Kate began facilitating organizational training and retreats after cofounding the Meditation Working Group at Occupy Wall Street in 2011. She went on to become a core faculty member of MIT's Presencing Institute and designed online political education programs for Buddhist Peace Fellowship. Currently, she works with leaders and organizations committed to sustainability and right relationships using awareness and embodiment practices to inform strategic planning and organizational culture.

Website: www.katejohnson.com

Instagram: @hellokatejohnson

Laura Khoudari is a pioneer in trauma-informed strength training; she is also a writer, speaker, wellness coach, and the author of the book *Lifting Heavy Things: Healing Trauma One Rep at a Time*. She uses her gift of storytelling in concert with her training and expertise to inspire and empower people to live fulfilling lives aligned with their own values, goals, interests, and strengths.

Her work has been widely recognized by the trauma and fitness community, and she has been featured in the *New York Times*, NPR, Buzzfeed, UpWorthy, Outside Online, Medium, Vice, and Nike.com. She has presented her work for Somatic Experiencing International, the Breathe Network, Reebok, Les Mills, Fitness4AllBodies, and conferences, schools, and fitness studios in the US and Canada.

Website: www.laurakhoudari.com

Instagram: @laurakhoudari

Eva Ludwig is a licensed psychotherapist with expertise in trauma (complex and developmental), attachment, relationships, and somatic integration. She earned a master's degree in social work from the University of Tennessee with a concentration in trauma treatment. Eva is fully trained in somatic and attachment-focused eye movement desensitization and reprocessing (EMDR) and uses all that she has learned about the body, Buddhism, and attachment in her integrative, person-centered approach.

Eva continues to explore the ways in which she can combine ancient healing and movement practices with modern modalities with the goal of inspiring and empowering clients. She pays special attention to healing intergenerational, complex, and developmental trauma in Black and Indigenous communities as well as other communities of color by employing a holistic whole-body approach so that they may be an igniting force of intergenerational healing.

Website: www.symmetry-counseling.com/eva-bio

Instagram: @evalinludwig

Dr. Sarah Mandel is a clinical psychologist who lives in New York City with her husband and two daughters. She received her doctorate in clinical psychology from Rutgers University. Prior to her stage-four cancer progression, she provided individual, couples, group, and family therapy in hospital, college counseling, and outpatient clinic settings throughout the New York City area. Her debut book, a memoir, is called *Little Earthquakes*.

Website: www.drsarahmandel.com

Lewis Mehl-Madrona, MD, graduated from Stanford University School of Medicine and trained in family medicine, psychiatry, and clinical psychology. He is interested in the relation of healing through dialogue in community and psychosis. He is the author of *Coyote Medicine*, *Coyote Healing*, and *Coyote Wisdom*, a trilogy of books on what Native culture has to offer the modern world. He has also written *Narrative Medicine, Healing the Mind through the Power of Story: The Promise of Narrative Psychiatry*, and, with Barbara Mainguy, *Remapping Your Mind: The Neuroscience of Self-Transformation through Story*. Lewis currently works with Wabanaki Public Health and Wellness, which serves the five tribes of Maine. He has been studying traditional healing and healers since his early days and has written about their work and the process of healing. His primary focus has been Cherokee and Lakota traditions, though he has also explored other Plains cultures and those of Northeastern North America. His goal is to bring the wisdom of Indigenous peoples about healing back into mainstream medicine and transform medicine and psychology through this wisdom coupled with more European-derived narrative traditions. He has written scientific papers in these areas and continues to do research. He writes an almost weekly blog on physical and mental health for www.future-health.org. His current interests center around psychosis and its treatment within community and with nonpharmacological means, narrative approaches to chronic pain and its use in primary care, and further developing healing paradigms within a narrative/Indigenous framework.

Website: www.mehl-madrona.com

Instagram: @mehlmadrona

Crystal McCreary is a lead yoga, mindfulness, health educator, and teacher trainer with thirteen-plus years of experience in instructing yoga and mindfulness to people of all ages. She is a coach and mentor with a passion for implementing comprehensive wellness programs within schools and organizations to foster compassionate and equitable communities and sustainable work environments. Crystal's expertise is derived from a lifetime of harnessing powerful, embodied, contemplative tools necessary to navigate the unique challenges of living as a Black girl and now ciswoman in an inequitable world. She facilitates training for many organizations that aim to support the social and emotional well-being of youth and adults, including the New York Department of Education, CUNY-Hunter Public Health Department, and mindful schools. She currently works full time on the health education team at the Dalton School in New York. Crystal has been featured in such publications as *Yoga Bodies*, *Mantra Yoga + Health* magazine, *Elephant*, *Yoga*, *Blavity*, the Shondaland.com blog, academic journals such as *Race and Yoga* (UC Berkeley), and numerous other blogs and podcasts. She graduated from Stanford University with a BA in African and African American studies, completed the American Conservatory Theater's master of fine arts program in acting, and is registered with the Yoga Alliance as a 500-ERYT and RCYT.

Website: crystalmccreary.com

Instagram: @crystalmccreary

Brenda Mitchell is the state chapter coleader for Moms Demand Action in Illinois and a fellow with the Everytown Survivor Network. In 2005, Brenda's thirty-one-year-old son, Kenneth, was shot and killed outside a sports bar one week after his younger brother, Kevin, left for his third tour of duty in Afghanistan. A single parent, Kenneth left behind three sons. Since her son's death, Brenda has become a dedicated advocate for gun violence prevention with an emphasis on trauma. An ordained pastor, she serves on the Everytown Faith Advisory Council; she is a complicated grief counselor and holds certification as a mindfulness counselor. In addition to her work with Everytown, she is an active member with the gun violence advocacy organization Purpose Over Pain, headquartered in Southside Chicago. She also has volunteered as a survivor on a committee with the Mayor's Office of Gun Violence Prevention.

Instagram: @bkmitchell1

Lori Meyers is a freelance writer who is passionate about her family and making life a little better for someone else every single day. After years as a grant writer, she turned her skills to writing nonfiction pieces about her life and commentary on life around her. Formerly a feature writer for the Lifestyle Magazine Group, she has been published in *Voices of Multiple Sclerosis* (LaChance Publishing, 2010).

Brette Popper teaches yoga, meditation, and breath-awareness techniques in New York City, where she leads group classes and sees students individually. A voracious student, she regularly studies Sanskrit, yoga philosophy, yoga therapy, and Buddhism to supplement her teaching and practice.

She was the founder of YogaCity NYC, the city's premier website for yoga news and information. In that role, she published, wrote, and acted as moderator for public panel discussions on topics of interest to the yoga community. Prior to her work in yoga, Brette sustained a career in magazine publishing for more than twenty years.

She served as president of *Quest Magazine*, a division of Meigher Communications, where she also acted as corporate vice president of business development. From 1985 until 1996, Brette worked for *USA Weekend*, a division of Gannett. For six years she served as president and publisher, performing the role of chief executive. She sits on the board of her co-op building and has worked closely with a variety of nonprofits, where she has headed boards and helped leaders achieve goals and develop strategies for growth.

Brette splits her time between New York City and Greece. She writes regularly for her newsletter and is working on her first book. Join Brette's newsletter, *Under the Surface*: tinyletter.com/Brette Popper.

Website: brettepopperyoga.com

Instagram: @brettepopper

Jillian Pransky, author of *Deep Listening*, is an international presenter and meditation teacher, and certified yoga therapist. She teaches at prominent wellness centers throughout the country and is the creator of Mindful of Rest: An Online Retreat and the Art of Conscious Rest: Restorative Yoga Teacher Training. A student of Pema Chödrön's work since 1998, Jillian infuses her yoga classes with mindfulness practices, compassion, and ease. For more than twenty-five years, Jillian has been teaching people all over the world the principles of deep listening, which sets conditions for personal awakening, community connections, and an integrative healing experience. Her message is simple but potent: slowing down, turning inward, and deeply listening to our bodies and hearts constitute perhaps the most meaningful form of self-care work we can do. When we are more compassionate and connected with ourselves, we are able to be more compassionate and connected with others and the world around us.

Website: www.jillianpransky.com

Instagram: @jillianpransky

La Sarmiento is an immigrant, nonbinary Filipinx-American. They were a retreat teacher with Tara Brach and the Guiding Teacher of the BIPOC and LGBTQIA+ Sanghas of the Insight Meditation Community of Washington. They are a 2012 graduate of the Spirit Rock Community Dharma Leaders Training Program and have also led mindfulness retreats for teens, young adults, women, and the LGBTQIA+ community around the United States. They are currently a mentor for the Mindfulness Meditation Teacher Certification Program and a teacher for Cloud Sangha. When they are not teaching, you'll find La singing dharma spoof songs with their ukulele; building with Legos; playing with their rescue pups, Annabel and Bader; baking a mean chocolate chip cookie; or kayaking or hiking with their life partner, Wendy.

Website: www.lasarmiento.com

Instagram: @bodhila

Julia Sedlock is a writer, designer, and community advocate based in the Hudson Valley. She is a partner of Cosmo Design Factory, a small practice that focuses on residential and community-based projects, and a founding member of several community organizations working on affordable housing and land stewardship in and around her home village of Philmont, New York.

She holds degrees in earth and environmental sciences, design criticism, and architecture, and her work explores relationality among the bodies, lands, buildings, and stories that we live within. She believes that these spaces, structures, and landscapes have the capacity to change us and, at their best, act as companions as we navigate our way through the stories of our lives. Her first book, *Creatures Are Stirring: A Guide to Architectural Companionship*, was coauthored with Joseph Altshuler and released by Applied Research and Design in 2022.

Instagram: @juliasedlock

Ann Tashi Slater has written for the *New Yorker*, the *Paris Review*, the *New York Times*, the *Washington Post, Guernica, Catapult, Tin House*, and *Granta*, among others, and she is a contributing editor at *Tricycle*. She speaks and teaches workshops in the US, Asia, and Europe, at the Rubin Museum of Art, the Asia Society, Princeton, Columbia, Oxford, and the American University of Paris. Based in Tokyo, she is working on a book about bardo and the art of living, and recently finished a memoir.

Website: www.anntashislater.com

Instagram: @anntashislater

Elizabeth L. Silver is the author of the novel *The Majority* (Riverhead, 2023), the memoir *The Tincture of Time: A Memoir of (Medical) Uncertainty* (Penguin, 2017), and the novel *The Execution of Noa P. Singleton* (Crown, 2013). Her work has been published in seven languages and optioned for film. Also an attorney, Elizabeth has written for the *Washington Post, New York Magazine, Harper's Bazaar*, and *McSweeney's* and currently teaches creative writing with the UCLA Writers Program. She is the founder and director of Onward Literary Mentoring and lives in Los Angeles with her family.

Website: www.elizabethlsilver.com
Instagram: @elizlsilver

Kim Thai (she/her) is an Emmy award–winning producer, writer, social justice advocate, and mindfulness teacher. She has shown President Biden the challenges of health-care workers; shot with Lizzo, Awkwafina, and Pete Davidson before they were big; and watched the rehearsal of Miley Cyrus's "Wrecking Ball" performance before it went viral. She is the founder of GaneshSpace, a mindfulness organization that creates healing spaces for historically excluded communities and social justice education for all, and the senior director of curriculum programming at Starts With Us, a growing movement to overcome the extreme cultural and political divides in America by leveraging media and technology to foster independent thinking and constructive communication across lines of difference.

She has studied yoga in India and taught the practice through an inclusive lens for more than five years; she has studied at the Trauma Resource Institute and looks at how oppression-based trauma can be released through somatic practices. She is currently studying nonviolence through the King Center, is a student in Thich Nhat Hanh's Plum Village tradition, and was given the dharma name Ancestral River of the Heart to widen and deepen the insight from Buddhist teachings. As a queer Asian woman and proud kid of Vietnamese refugees, her personal mission is to empower people with liberatory practices to live with ease and joy.

Website: www.thekimthai.com
Instagram: @kthai6

Shelly Tygielski is the author *of Sit Down to Rise Up: How Radical Self-Care Can Change the World*. She is the founder of Pandemic of Love, a global grassroots mutual aid community that has directly matched nearly three million people with supporters since the beginning of the COVID-19 pandemic in March 2020, accounting for more than $100 million in direct transactions. Her work has been featured in more than one hundred media outlets, including CNN Heroes (2020), *Forbes*, Upworthy, *The Kelly Clarkson Show*, *CBS This Morning*, the *New York Times*, and the *Washington Post*. Shelly has been praised by individuals from President Joe Biden to Arianna Huffington and Dr. Jon Kabat-Zinn to Maria Shriver. She is a trauma-informed mindfulness teacher named one of the 12 Powerful Women of the Mindfulness Movement by *Mindful Magazine* in 2019. Shelly teaches formalized self-care and resilience practices at organizations around the world and is widely regarded as a self-care activist.

Website: www.shellytygielski.com

Instagram: @mindfulskatergirl

Jamia Wilson is an award-winning feminist activist, writer, speaker, and podcaster. She joined Penguin Random House as vice president and executive editor in 2021. As the former director of the Feminist Press at the City University of New York and the former VP of programs at the Women's Media Center, Jamia has been a leading voice on women's rights issues for over a decade. Her work has appeared in numerous outlets, including the *New York Times*, the *Today Show*, CNN, *Elle*, BBC, *Rookie*, *Refinery 29*, *Glamour*, *Teen Vogue*, and the *Washington Post*. She is the author of *This Book Is Feminist*; *Young, Gifted, and Black*; the introduction and oral history in *Together We Rise: Behind the Scenes at the Protest Heard Around the World*; *Step into Your Power: 23 Lessons on How to Live Your Best Life*; *Big Ideas for Young Thinkers*; and *The ABCs of AOC*. She is the coauthor of *Road Map for Revolutionaries: Resistance, Advocacy, and Activism for All*. Jamia is passionate about mission-driven organizations and serves on the board for the Omega Institute, Feminist.com, and the Center for Reproductive Rights boards, as well as the St. Timothy's School

Advisory Council. She is also the cohost of the second season of the Anthem Award–winning podcast *Ordinary Equality*.

Website: www.jamiawilson.com

Instagram: @jamiaawilson

Carla Zanoni is a poet and author who is writing her first book, a memoir on self-worth. She is an award-winning journalist, writer, poet, and media strategist, and she was the first Latina named to the *Wall Street Journal*'s masthead. She is also TED's first head of audience development. Originally from Argentina, Carla grew up in New Jersey and now splits her time between the hills of Upper Manhattan in New York City and the mountains of the northern Catskills in New York State. You can subscribe to her newsletter *The Em Dash* at carla.substack.com.

Website: www.carlazanoni.com

Instagram: @carlazanoni

Meghan Zipin is a poet and mama who shares her time writing with discovering half-eaten snacks around the house and ensuring her children stay little for as long as possible. Meghan's writing asks readers to feel something in their body and look at the world with a tender set of eyes. Her first book, *First Light*, a poetry collection chronicling her survival of the Boston Marathon bombing, her life with PTSD, and her love of motherhood, was published in April 2023. She lives on eleven acres in New Hampshire with her husband, three curly-haired boys, and their dog, Oona.

Website: www.meghanzipin.com

Instagram: @mismegs82

Notes

1. Peter Levine, *Healing Trauma: Restoring the Wisdom of the Body* (Sounds True, 2008).
2. B. K. S. Iyengar, *Sparks of Divinity: The Teachings of B. K. S. Iyengar* (Shambhala, 2012).
3. Resmaa Menakem, *My Grandmother's Hands* (Central Recovery, 2017).
4. Antonia Mufarach, "The Stories We Tell About Ourselves: Understanding Our Personal Narratives with Psychologist Dan McAdams," *North by Northwestern*, January 25, 2022, https://northbynorthwestern.com/the-stories-we-tell-about-ourselves/.
5. Chimamanda Ngozi Adichie, *We Should All Be Feminists* (Vintage Books, 2015), 27.
6. William Faulkner, *Requiem for a Nun* (Random House, 1951).
7. Tricia Hersey, "Rest Is Anything That Connects Your Mind and Body," *Nap Ministry* (blog), February 21, 2022, https://thenapministry.wordpress.com/2022/02/21/rest-is-anything-that-connects-your-mind-and-body/.
8. Joy Harjo, *An American Sunrise* (W. W. Norton, 2019).
9. Lewis Mehl Madrona, *Coyote Wisdom: The Power of Story in Healing* (Bear, 2005).
10. Krista Tippett, *Becoming Wise: An Inquiry to the Mystery and Art of Living* (Penguin, 2016), 29.

11. Ethan Nichtern, *The Road Home* (North Point Press, 2016).

12. Sharon Salzberg, *Lovingkindness: The Revolutionary Art of Happiness* (Shambhala, 2018).

13. Pema Chodron, *Start Where You Are: A Guide to Compassionate Living* (Shambhala, 2004).

14. Parker Palmer, *Let Your Life Speak: Listening for the Voice of Vocation* (Jossey-Bass, 2000), 7–8.

15. Octavia E. Butler, "How I Built Novels Out of Writer's Blocks," *Writer's Digest*, June 1999.

16. Tarana Burke, *Unbound: My Story of Liberation and the Birth of the Me Too Movement* (Flatiron Books, 2021).

17. Virginia Woolf, *The Waves* (Penguin UK, 2019).

18. Rebecca Solnit, *The Faraway Nearby* (Penguin, 2013), 60.

19. Lewis Mehl Madrona, *Coyote Healing: Miracles in Native Medicine* (Bear, 2003).

20. James Gordon, *The Transformation: Discovering Wholeness and Healing After Trauma* (HarperOne, 2019).

21. Stephen W. Porges, *The Pocket Guide to the Polyvagal Theory: The Transformative Power of Feeling Safe* (W. W. Norton, 2017).

22. Rachel Naomi Remen, *Kitchen Table Wisdom: Stories That Heal, 10th Anniversary Edition* (Penguin, 2006), 144.

23. Molly Young, "Out Loud, Pumped Up and Bossed Around by the French," *New York Times*, November 5, 2022.

24. University of South Australia, "Reading Builds Resilience Among At-Risk Kids," *Science Daily*, March 8, 2022, https://www.sciencedaily.com/releases/2022/03/220308102826.htm.

25. Greg J. Stephens, Lauren J. Silbert, and Uri Hasson, "Speaker-Listener Neural Coupling Underlies Successful Communication," *Proceedings of the National Academy of Sciences of the United States of America* 107, no. 32 (2010): 14425–14430, https://10.1073/pnas.1008662107.

26. Uri Hasson, Asif A. Ghazanfar, Bruno Galantucci, Simon Garrod, and Christian Keysers, "Brain-to-Brain Coupling: A

Mechanism for Creating and Sharing a Social World," *Trends in Cognitive Sciences* 16, no. 2 (2012): 114–121, https://doi.org/10.1016/j.tics.2011.12.007.

27. Haruki Murakami, *Kafka on the Shore* (Knopf Doubleday, 2006), 51.

28. Melissa Febos, *Body Work: The Radical Power of Personal Narrative* (Manchester University Press, 2022).

29. Joan Didion, *The White Album* (Simon and Schuster, 1979).

30. Thich Nhat Hanh, *Walking Meditation* (Sounds True, 2006).

Index

240–241; listening with love and, 242–243; music and, 137–138; sound meditation, 77–78; two-way writing practice, 174
literary citizenship, 277
Ludwig, Eva, 13, 104

Madrona, Lewis Mehl, 214–215
Mandel, Sarah, 98–99
McAdams, Dan, 14
McCreary, Crystal, 6–8, 14–15
Me Too movement, 121
medicine, 70, 171
meditation practice, xxiv, 23–24, 73–74, 77–78, 81–82, 280–281. *See also* mindfulness
Mellk, Julie, 89
memories: narrative therapy and, 98–99; returning the happy, 101–102; trauma and, xxvii–xxviii; writing exercises and, 142
Metta meditation, 81–82
Meyers, Lori, 260–262
Mind Body Institute (Harvard), 10
mindfulness, 59, 96–97, 183, 238–239. *See also* meditation
mindfulness meditation, 23–24
Missing Piece (Silverstein), 179
Mitchell, Brenda, 112–113
Morrison, Toni, 61
motherhood, 272–273
music, 88, 137–138

Narrative Healing, xxiii–xxv, xix–xxx, 251–252
narrative therapy, 98–99

natural cycles, 72
nature, 236
neck, 39, 231–232
nervous system, 12–14, 58–60, 200–202
Nichtern, Ethan, 73

obstacles, 103, 105, 163–164
Oliver, Mary, 111

pain, 127–128, 147, 253, 260–262
Palmer, Parker, 91
physical exercises: body scan, 63–64; chest/heart expansion, 43–44; expanding, 34–35; feeling support of the earth, 32; finding your seat, 20; foot sensitivity and, 21–22; grief pressure point and, 40; "handshake" practice, 30–31; for the heart, 203–204; hug, 154; lifting legs, 45; moving off balance, 186; relaxation, 39; releasing trauma, 29; rest, 46–47; shaking exercises, 41, 141; side lean, 271; taking up space/mountain pose, 26–27; tapping, 115–116; twist to support digestion, 79–80; warming up, 19; for wrists, 33
plants, 236
playfulness, 259
polyvagal theory (PVT), 201–202
Popper, Brette, 175–176
Porges, Stephen, 202
PostSecret, 187
posture, 267
"Power and Time" (Oliver), 111
power differentials, 104

Pransky, Jillian, 193–197
publishing, 270

Qigong shaking, 6, 41

readers, 130, 268–269
reading, 83, 131, 189, 223
recovery, xx, 6
Relaxation Response, The (Benson), 62
religion, 265–266
remembered wellness, 101–102
resilience, 136
rest, 46–47, 218, 264
Road Home, The (Nichtern), 73

safe listeners, 212–213
safe places, 173
Salzberg, Sharon, 81–82
Sarmiento, La, 257–259
scalp, 39
seat, 20
secrets, 187–188
Sedlock, Julia, 180
sensations, 8, 12
service, 277, 279
sexual assault, 121, 253
shame, 5, 198, 200, 264
Shapiro, Dani, 95
silence, 67–69
Silver, Elizabeth L., 208–209
Slater, Ann Tashi, 270
slowing down, 28
sound meditation, 77–78
speaking, 205
stories: ancestors and, 65–66; author's, 194–197; of breath, 120; buried in body, 8–10; communicating with whole

body, 263; healing and, 251–254; hero's journey and, 150; identities and, 257–259; importance of listening to the whole, 214–215; letting go of, 233–234; needs of, 129; nervous system and, 12–14; observed, 235; one-on-one sharing of, 199–200; pain and, 127–128, 260–262; as particles, 175–176; personification of, 152; planning, 180–181; recurring, 122; releasing of to listen, 58–59; resistance and, 258–259; rewriting, 114; sense of safety and, 14; sharing with another, xxv, 194–200; social change, 252; timing/method of telling, 208–209; transformation and, 198–199, 252–255; yoga practice and discovery of, 14–15
support systems, 212

technology, 206–207
tension, 39, 48
Thai, Kim, 56, 65, 103
"thinking position," 11
throat, 231–232
tightrope walking, 160–162
Tippet, Krista, 71
Tonglen practice, 85–86
transformation, 198–199, 252–255
Transformation, The (Gordon), 200
trauma: creating a safe place and, 173; isolation and, 32; mind-body connection and, xxvii, 7–8; new narratives and, 112–113; one-on-one relationships and,